Stoic Book of Anger 1

SENECA ON ANGER
CAUSES AND CONSEQUENCES

Dr. Chuck Chakrapani

The Stoic Gym Publications

Gratitude
Cover design
Kumiko Yoshida
Cover image
Nero and Seneca, by Eduardo Barrón (1904). Museo del Prado. Licensed under Creative Commons.
Copy edits
Nancy Kramarch
Gail Seymour

The Stoic Gym Publications
www.TheStoicGym.Com

Stoic Books of Anger Volume 1/ Chuck Chakrapani. —1st ed.
ISBN 978-0-920219-73-7 (Print); 978-0-920219-74-4 (ebook)

Contents

SENECA'S 'ON ANGER' . BOOK TWO
ANGER. A DELIBERATE CHOICE
WHAT TO DO ABOUT IT

INTRODUCTION

Seneca 'On Anger'

Who was Seneca?

Lucius Annaeus Seneca, or Seneca the Younger, was a Stoic philosopher. Born around 4 BCE in Cordoba in Spain and raised in Rome, he became an orator. While in Rome, Seneca made a persuasive speech which aroused the Emperor Caligula's jealousy. Caligula spared Seneca's life only because he believed Seneca would die soon.

The reprieve did not last long. Messalina, the wife of the next emperor, Claudius, accused Seneca of committing adultery with the Emperor's niece, Julia Livilla, and had him banished in 41 CE.

Several years later, Seneca was invited back to Rome by Nero's mother and became first a tutor to Nero and then his advisor. Because of his position, he lived well. Most likely, he was the richest man in Rome at that time, probably a billionaire by today's standards. Seneca was not only a Stoic philosopher but a statesman, dramatist, and humorist.

When he was 66 years old, Seneca requested an audience with Nero and sought to be relieved of his public duties due to his old age. Seneca then quietly retired to his country estates, seldom visiting Rome.

Three years later, when he was 69 years old, Nero accused Seneca of being involved in a plot to kill the emperor and ordered Seneca to kill himself. So he did.

What is *On Anger*?

On Anger, initially written in Latin (*De Ira*) by Seneca, is a set of three books describing the causes and consequences of anger and how to avoid them. Although Seneca was probably the richest man in the Roman empire, he was subject to the whims of three successive emperors. He incurred the wrath of Caligula, was exiled by Claudius, and was forced to commit suicide by Nero.

Although it is believed to be based on Chrysippus' work, *On Anger* is a distinct work written with conviction. It may well be one of the best books ever written on anger management.

Seneca addresses *On Anger* to his brother Novatus (who changed the name to Gallio later). However, it is more likely that he wrote it for posterity, as did his *Epistulae Morales*.

What is "the plain English version"?

This is a plain English version of *On Anger*. The most important reason for a plain English version is that the standard translations have an implicit obligation to follow the original text carefully.

Unfortunately, the original text was written more than two thousand years ago in Latin. In the intervening time, the meaning of words, phrases, and idioms have changed.

All this creates problems for the modern reader. Mostly, the standard translations look daunting. I found that the translations, as excellent as they might be, were not easy to read for several reasons such as:

- Dense layouts;
- Archaic and intrusive numbering systems;
- Convoluted sentences; and
- No headings or subheadings to guide the reader.

These may not deter scholars and academics, but common readers may not be so motivated. It is not the fault of the translators either. After all, translators are bound by the structure of the original text written about two thousand years ago. In general, they cannot deviate from it, even if the translation gets obscure in places. They can add footnotes and explanations, but that calls for additional effort to understand.

A reader who is not reading *On Anger* for scholarly purposes can benefit immensely from a rendition that is true to the intent of the original text but uses contemporary English. This is what this edition of *On Anger* does. More specifically, this edition:

- Uses modern English, simple words, and shorter sentences.
- Rearranges a few sentences so they flow well.
- Attempts to use gender-neutral language when the principles are clearly applicable to both men and women. (However, when Seneca occasionally uses sexist language, I left it as is. I didn't 'sanitize' his writings.)

I have also introduced some enhancements to the original:

- Descriptive titles and subheadings.
- A summary of the key ideas of each chapter at the beginning.

Through all these changes, I have tried to remain faithful to the spirit of what Seneca was trying to say. To this end, I consulted several translations by eminent scholars while putting this edition together.

Is there a cost to all these changes?

Probably.

There might be some occasional loss in accuracy, mainly when used for scholarly purposes—as can happen when a legal document is written in plain English.

But I believe the benefits of readability far outweigh the disadvantages of minor inaccuracies in places. Saki put it so well, "A little inaccuracy sometimes maybe saves tons of explanation."

Is this book for you?

If you aim to understand Seneca's *On Anger* without spending too much time and effort, you have come to the right place. If you are looking for a scholarly translation of *On Anger,* perhaps you should look elsewhere.

BASIC IDEAS

Anger: Its Causes and Consequences

Seneca's first two books *On Anger* (covered in this volume) deals with the following themes:

Anger is destructive

Anger, in all its forms, is more devastating than any plague. It destroys our reason and causes considerable damage. Both individuals and countries are destroyed by anger. Anger is mad because it is bent on hurting others, even though doing so will also hurt the angry person.

Anger serves no useful purpose

Anger serves no useful purpose. Our weakness causes it, and it is poison. However, we should not be mad at those who are angry with us because it will destroy us. Even if we have to punish someone, we should not do it in anger. Because it serves no useful purpose, we should completely eliminate anger from our lives.

Anger is a choice

Even though it may seem that we are helplessly driven by rage, anger is our choice. It cannot happen without our assent. Therefore, we can learn not to be angry. Anger is curable and even avoidable.

We can avoid anger

Anger is a sliding slope. Once we give in to anger, we quickly lose control. So, it is best to avoid getting angry in the first place. We can do this by not being credulous, seeing through irrational anger, not living too soft a life, delaying the onset of anger, and avoiding our impulse to avenge any perceived injury. It will also help us if we don't take on too much, associate ourselves with peaceful people, and make it a rule not to act when we are angry. Changing our physical expressions of anger can also soften or eliminate it.

We can manage anger

Once we are angry, we can use several strategies to manage anger such as seeing things from the other person's perspective, not persisting in our anger even if it is justified, not comparing ourselves with others, being grateful for what we have, ignoring trifles, and understanding how money causes anger. We can also see how we will be dead soon and realize that it is futile to waste our lives by being angry.

SENECA'S "ON ANGER." BOOK 1

ANGER, A SLIDING SLOPE

CHAPTER 1

Anger is Temporary Madness

Key ideas of this chapter

1. *The angry are thirsty for revenge even though it hurts them as well.*
2. *Anger is temporary madness. Those who are angry resemble the insane.*
3. *The signs of anger are ugly, and we cannot conceal it.*

The importance of softening our anger

Novatus, you asked me to write about anger, and how we may soften it. I think you are right to be terrified of this ugliest and most brutal of all emotions. Other passions have some degree of peace and quiet. But anger is all action. It explodes the impulse of grief with an inhuman desire for weapons, blood, and torture. It doesn't care as long as it hurts another. It is greedy for revenge even when it drags down the avenger along with it.

Anger is a brief madness

Some wise people have, therefore, called anger a fleeting madness. It has no self-control, doesn't care for dignity, forgets friendships, and is tenacious in finishing what it started, all in equal measure. It is deaf to reason and advice, excited by minor things, and unable to see what is real and just. It is like a falling rock that breaks into pieces when it falls on the item it crushes.

Anger changes our looks

To understand that people who are in the grips of anger are not sane, watch how they look.

Here are the unmistakable signs that identify the mad:

- aggressive and threatening expressions
- knitted brows
- wrinkled faces
- tense walks
- nervous hands
- different skin colors
- quick and heavy breathing

The same signs identify an angry person too:

- their eyes burn and shine
- their whole face turns red with the boiling blood that rushes from the bottom of their heart
- their lips quiver
- their teeth clench
- their hair bristles and stands on end

- their breath is labored and hissing
- their joints crack as they twist them
- they groan and burst into gibberish

They often clap their hands together and stamp their feet. Their whole body is agitated and plays tricks that reveal a disturbed mind.

Thus, it provides us with an ugly and shocking picture of self-parody and excitement. You cannot tell what describes this better: unpleasant or disgusting.

We cannot conceal anger

Other things can be hidden away and secretly cherished. But anger announces itself openly and "in your face." The more intense it is, the more plainly it boils forth. Don't you see how, in all animals, specific signals appear when they are about to attack? And how their entire body gives up their usual calm appearance as ferocity takes over?

Boars foam at the mouth and sharpen their teeth by rubbing them against trees; bulls toss their horns in the air and scatter the sand with their hooves; lions roar; enraged snakes puff up their necks; mad dogs look sullen. There is no animal so fearsome and noxious by nature that, when seized by anger, it does not become even more so.

I am fully aware that other passions, such as lust, fear, and courage, are also hard to hide. They, too, give signs of their presence and can be discovered in advance. There is no intense passion that does not change our appearance.

Then what's the difference between such emotions and anger?

For other passions, the signs are visible; for anger, they prominently stand out.

Think about this

[Anger] is like a falling rock that breaks into pieces when it falls on the thing it crushes.

CHAPTER 2

Anger Causes Great Damage

Key points of this chapter

1. *Anger has done more significant damage to humankind than any plague.*
2. *Both individuals and communities are destroyed by it.*
3. *Even a semblance of anger is enough to cause damage.*

No plague has done greater harm

If you want to examine the results of anger and the damage it causes, I say that no plague has done greater harm to humankind.

You will see slaughter and poisons, accusations and counteraccusations, destruction of cities, the ruin of whole groups of people, auctioning of prominent people [presumably prisoners of war], torching of houses. The flames are not confined within city walls but make the entire country glow with the enemy flame.

Individuals are destroyed by anger

Look at the foundations of the most famous cities. They are hardly visible now. Anger ruined them.

Look at the deserts that extend for many miles without anyone living there. They were made barren by anger.

Look at leaders who are cited as unfortunate. Anger stabbed one of them in his own bed, struck down another even though rules of hospitality protected him, tore another one to pieces in a court as a crowded forum watched, ordered yet another to shed to his blood as his son killed him. Anger ordered a royal to have his neck cut by a slave and another to have his limb stretch out on the cross.

Communities destroyed by anger

So far, I have been talking only about individual cases.

What if you were to go beyond individuals destroyed by anger and consider communities cut down by the sword, people butchered by soldiers sent against them, and entire countries condemned to death through indiscriminate slaughter?

Why are people angry with a gladiator, and so unjust as to get upset if he does not die cheerfully? They think they are scorned. They show by their looks, gestures, and excitement that they have turned from being just a spectator into an adversary.

Even a semblance of anger causes destruction

Everything of this sort is not anger, but they resemble anger. Like children who want to beat the ground they fall upon, they often do not even know why they are angry. They are angry without any reason and without having been injured in any way. Yet they have a sense of injury and would like to exact a penalty for it.

They are deceived by the likeness of blows and are appeased by the pretended tears of those who despise their anger. Thus, an act of unreal revenge heals unreal grief.

Think about this

If you want to examine the results of anger and the damage it causes, I say that no plague has done more significant harm to humankind.

CHAPTER 3

Anger Drives Out Reason

Key points of this chapter

1. *Sometimes we get angry in anticipation of an injury.*
2. *Even the most powerless person can injure a powerful person.*
3. *Animals may appear angry. But their quality of anger is different because they cannot reason. Anger is uniquely human.*
4. *Anger is the enemy of reason, and it does not arise in places where reason prevails.*

Even the weakest can hurt the powerful

Our challenger says, "We often are angry not with those who have hurt us, but with those who are going to hurt us. So you may be sure that anger is not born of injury."

We are indeed angry with those who are going to hurt us. But they already have harmed us in intention. One intends to do an injury is already doing it.

Our challenger argues, "The weakest are often angry with the strongest. So, you may be sure that anger is not a desire to punish their rival. People do not desire to punish those who they cannot hope to punish."

In the first place, I spoke of a desire to inflict punishment, not the power to do so. People desire things even when they cannot get them.

In the next place, no one is so low in status as not to be able to hope to inflict punishment even upon the greatest of men. We all are powerful to carry out some mischief.

Animals don't feel emotions the same way as humans

Aristotle's definition differs little from mine. He says that anger is a desire to repay suffering. It would take a while to examine the differences between his description and mine.

Both of us can be persuaded that wild animals become angry without being offended by injury, and without having any idea of punishing or avenging. Even though they do these things, these are not what they intend to do. We must admit that wild animals and other creatures except human beings are not subject to anger.

Anger is the enemy of reason

Anger is the enemy of reason, and it does not live in places where reason lives. Wild animals have impulses, fury, cruelty, aggressiveness. But they don't have anger any more than they have luxury. They do indulge in some pleasures with less self-control than human beings. Do not believe the poet who says:

> *The boar his wrath forgets, the stag forgets the hounds,*
> *The bear forgets how 'midst the herd he leaped with frantic bounds.*

Only human beings get angry

When he speaks of animals being angry, he means that they are excited and provoked. They don't know how to be angry any more they know how to pardon.

Dumb creatures don't have human feelings but have certain impulses that resemble them. If they could feel love and hate, they would also be capable of friendship and enmity, of disagreement and agreement. Although some traces of these qualities exist even in them, conditions like good and bad belong only to human beings.

Only humans have been given wisdom, foresight, industry, and reflection. Animals are not given human virtues or vices. Their entire constitution, mental and physical, is unlike that of human beings. Their royal and leading principle is drawn from another source.

They possess a voice, yet not a clear one, but indistinct and incapable of forming words. They have a tongue, but one which is constrained, not agile enough to produce complex sounds. And they possess intellect, the greatest attribute of all, but it is crude and imprecise.

As a result, they can grasp those visions and fragments which stir them to action but only in a hazy and blurry fashion. Consequently, their impulses and outbreaks are violent, and they do not feel fear, anxiety, grief, or anger, but some semblances of these feelings.

Therefore, they quickly drop them and adopt the opposite. They graze after showing the most intense rage and terror and fall into quiet sleep after frantic bellowing and plunging.

This about this

Anger is the enemy of reason, and it does not live in places where reason lives.

CHAPTER 4

Anger Comes in Many Forms

Key points of this chapter

1. *Anger comes in many forms and is described using many words: bitter, harsh, peevish, frantic, loud, rude, and fierce, and so on.*
2. *Anger is evil in all its thousand names.*

Being angry vs. being quick-tempered

I explained sufficiently what anger is. The difference between being angry and being quick-tempered is clear. It is the same as the difference between a drunken man and a drunkard, between a frightened man and a coward. An angry man not to be quick-tempered; a quick-tempered may sometimes not get mad.

Anger's many forms

I will skip the other kinds of anger that the Greeks have names for because we have no unique words for them in our language. Although we call people bitter, harsh, peevish, frantic, loud, rude, and fierce, they are all different forms being quick-tempered. You can add to this list sulkiness, a refined way of being quick-tempered. Some types of anger go no further than noise, while some are as lasting as they are common. Some are fierce in action but not so in words. Some are expressed in bitter terms and curses. Some do not go beyond complaining and turning one's back. Some are great, deep-seated, and brood within a person. There are a thousand other forms of this evil.

Think about this

There are a thousand different forms of this evil [anger]

.

CHAPTER 5

Anger is Incompatible with Nature

The key point of this chapter

Humankind is born for mutual assistance, anger for mutual ruin. Therefore, anger is incompatible with nature.

We have now completed our inquiry as to what anger is, whether it exists in any other animal besides us, what the difference is between it and being quick-tempered, and how many forms it has.

Is anger in accordance with nature?

Let us now enquire whether anger is in accordance with nature and whether it is useful and worthwhile to some extent.

Whether it is according to nature will become clear if we consider human nature. What is more gentle than human nature when it is in its proper condition? Yet, what is crueler than anger? What is more affectionate to others than a human being? Yet, what is more brutal against them than anger?

Humankind is born for mutual assistance, anger for mutual ruin. Humans love society, anger alienation. The one loves to do good, the other to harm, the one to help even strangers, the other to attack even its dearest friends. The one is ready yet to sacrifice itself for the good of others, the other to plunge into danger provided it drags others with it.

Anger is incompatible with nature

Who, then, can be more ignorant of nature than one who groups this cruel and hurtful vice as belonging to nature's best and most polished work? Anger, as we have said, is eager to punish. That such a desire should exist in a person's peaceful heart is least of all according to their nature. Human life is founded on benefits and harmony and is bound together into a partnership for the collective help of all. Not by terror, but by love towards one another.

Think about this

Human life is founded on benefits and harmony and is bound together into a partnership for the common help of all. Not by terror, but by love towards one another.

CHAPTER 6

Why Anger is Incompatible with Nature

Key points of this chapter

1. *Sometimes punishment is necessary. But, as with doctors, law administrators give out harsh penalties only as a last resort.*
2. *Human nature does not wish to punish. But anger wants to punish. Therefore, it is not compatible with human nature.*

What about punishment?

"What, then? Is not correction sometimes necessary?" Of course, it is—but with caution, not with anger. Caution does not injure; it heals under the guise of injury. We scorch crooked spears to straighten them and force them by driving in wedges. We do this not to break but to take the bends out of them. In the same way, we apply pain to the body or mind to correct traits made crooked by vice.

A physician treats gently, as far as possible

The physician, when dealing with slight illnesses, at first tries not to make much change in her patient's daily habits, to regulate his food, drink, and exercise. Instead, she works to improve the health of the patient just by changing the order in which he takes them.

Next, she changes the amount of each. If neither changing the order nor changing the amount works, she drops some and reduces others. If even this does not work, she bans eating altogether to make the body lighter.

If milder remedies don't work, only then does she open a vein, and if the extremities are injuring the body and infecting it with a disease, she deals with the limbs. Yet none of this treatment is considered harsh if its purpose is to give health.

An administrator is not eager to punish

Similarly, it is the duty of those who administer the laws to correct hostile people with words as much as possible. He may use gentle words to persuade them to do the right thing, inspire them with a love of honor and justice, and cause them to hate vice and place value upon virtue.

He should then use more persuasive language but continue advising and reprimanding. He must resort to punishments only in extreme cases, still making the sanctions mild and temporary.

He should reserve severe penalties only for outrageous crimes, making sure that no one dies, even if the criminal thinks he should die.

Law administrators differ from physicians on only one point. Physicians make it easy for patients to die if they cannot possibly help them live while law administrators attach shame and disgrace to the condemned.

They don't do this because they take pleasure in punishing anyone. The wise are far from such inhuman viciousness. They do it as a warning to others and, because the condemned were not useful to the state when alive, it may at least profit from their death.

Human nature does not wish to punish

Human nature does not want to punish. Therefore, anger is not in accordance with human nature because anger intends to punish. I will also cite Plato's argument: what's the harm in using others' arguments if they are on our side?

"A good person," says he, "does not hurt; it is the punishment that hurts. Punishment, therefore, is not consistent with a good person."

Neither is anger because they are compatible with each other. If a good person takes no pleasure in punishment, neither will they have a state of mind that delights in punishment.

Therefore, anger is not natural to human beings.

Think about this

Human nature does not wish to punish. Thus, anger is not in accordance with human nature.

CHAPTER 7

Anger Takes Over Once Let In

Key points of this chapter

1. *Because anger motivates and energizes us, it would appear that it could be a useful emotion.*
2. *However, there are at least two reasons why we should avoid anger altogether.*
   a. *It is easier not to let in anger than to let it in and try to control it.*
   b. *Reason can keep anger at bay. But once reason mixes with anger, it won't be able to restrain it.*

Isn't anger useful sometimes?

Even if anger is unnatural, shouldn't we adopt it because it may prove useful? It lifts the spirit and energizes it. Without it, courage cannot achieve anything significant in war. The fire is not lit unless its flame comes from this source. It is the prod that provokes the bold and sends them to face danger.

Therefore, some consider it best to moderate anger, rather than to get rid of it entirely; to control its excesses, and force it to keep within limits; to retain that part of it without which action will become slow and all mental strength and energy will be depleted.

Reasons against

First, it is easier not to admit harmful emotions than to control them. Once they are accepted, they take control of our minds. They are more robust than our lawful ruler (reason), and they will not allow themselves to be weakened or diminished.

Second, reason, which holds the reins, is only compelling as long as we keep it away from passion. If it mixes with passion and contaminates itself, it will not be able to restrain those whom it could have removed from its path. The mind, once excited and shaken, goes where passions drive it.

Certain things are under our power at the beginning. But, as they develop, they drag us along by their momentum and do not allow us to pull back. Those who have thrown themselves over a cliff have no control over their movements, and they cannot stop or slacken their pace. Once started, the unstoppable fall cuts off every thought and regret. They cannot help arriving at a place they could have avoided.

The mind, once it gives itself to anger, love, or any other passion, has no chance to check its momentum. Its weight and the downward slide of vices get hold of it and pull it down to the bottom.

Think about this

It is easier not to admit harmful emotions than to control them. Once we admit them, they take control of our minds.

CHAPTER 8

Anger and Reason Don't Mix

Key points of this chapter

1. *We should reject the first stirrings of anger. We should keep anger as far away as possible.*
2. *Reason is stronger than passion. But reason can defeat passion only if we don't mix them.*
3. *The angry are never ruled by reason, even though at times it might seem so.*

Reject the first stirrings of anger

It is best to reject straight away the first inducements to anger, to resist it from the very beginning, and to take care not to be drawn into it. Once it starts carrying us away, it is hard to get back again into a healthy condition. Reason counts for nothing once we admit passion into our mind, and voluntarily give it a certain authority. From then on, it will do whatever it pleases, not what we allow it to do.

No, the enemy must be met as far as away as possible and driven back. Once it enters the city through its gates, it will not allow its prisoners to set bounds to its victory.

The mind can no more stand aside, watching the passions to stop their advance. The mind itself, now weakened and misapplied, turns into a passion. It is unable to recover its helpful and healthy strength.

Passion and reason don't have designated places

Passion and reason, as I said before, don't have distinct provinces. Rather the mind itself changes for better or for worse. How then can reason recover when it has given way to anger and is defeated and held down by vices? How can it free itself from a confused mixture of mostly the lower qualities?

"But," argues our challenger, "some angry people control themselves."

Can they control themselves so completely that they do nothing which anger asks of them, or only somewhat? If [they control themselves so completely that they do] nothing, it is clear that anger is not needed, although your group said that anger has greater strength than reason. [It is not clear here what "group" the "challenger" belongs to.]

Reason is stronger than anger

Finally, I ask, is anger stronger or weaker than reason? If stronger, how can reason check it, since only the less powerful obey? If weaker, then reason can achieve its goals without anger and does not need the help of a less powerful quality.

Reason does not rule the angry

"But some angry people remain consistent and control themselves."

When do they do so? It is only when their anger disappears and voluntarily leaves. When it was red-hot, it was more powerful than them.

"So what? Don't they, even when very angry, sometimes let their enemies go unhurt and whole?"

They do. But when do they do it? Only when one passion overpowers another. When either fear or greed gets the upper hand, it is not because of reason that anger is subdued. It is due to an untrustworthy and temporary truce between the passions.

Think about this

It is best to reject right away the first inducements to anger, to resist it from the very beginning, and to take care not to be drawn into it.

CHAPTER 9

Anger Serves No Useful Purpose

Key points of this chapter

1. *Anger is useless. One can accomplish everything, including going to war without becoming angry.*
2. *When people go to war or punish others, if they don't do so out of eagerness, but because it is the right thing to do, then it is not anger.*
3. *Passions don't know how to obey or command.*

Anger does not stir the mind to right actions

Anger has no use. It does not stir the mind to brave actions. A virtue is self-sufficient and does not need the help of a vice. [A bold step does not need the support of anger.]

When virtue needs energy to act, it does not become angry, but rises to the occasion. It energizes or relaxes as required, just as the tension of dart machines that may be increased at the manager's pleasure.

Aristotle was wrong in believing otherwise

"Anger," says Aristotle, "is necessary, nor can any fight be won without it, unless it fills the mind, and kindles up the spirit. It must, however, be made use of, not as a general, but as a soldier."

This is not true.

Understanding the nature of anger

If anger listens to reason and follows its leads, it is no longer anger, because anger is stubborn. If it is disobedient and will not be quiet when ordered but is carried away by its own intentional and impulsive spirit, it is then useless and cannot help the mind. It is like a soldier who disregards a general's signal to retreat.

I understand that anger is unrestrained and unmanageable. Therefore, if anger allows limits to be imposed upon it, it ceases to be anger and must be called by a different name.

If it does not allow restrictions to be imposed upon it, it is harmful and cannot be considered helpful.

Therefore, either it is not anger, or it is useless.

If anyone wants to punish because it is the right thing to do and not because they are eager to punish, then that person is not angry but a useful soldier who knows how to obey. Passions don't know how to obey or how to command.

Think about this

Passions don't know how to obey or how to command.

CHAPTER 10

Reason Doesn't Seek Help from Passion

Key points of this chapter

1. *The mind can find no rest in passion.*
2. *Reason will never seek the help of passion and does not need its help.*

Reason will never seek the help of passion

Because [passions can neither obey nor command], reason will never seek the help of such blind and fierce impulses. If reason has no power over passions, it cannot control them except by using equally powerful passions: fear against anger, anger against idleness, greed against cowardice. Virtue seeking help from vice? Let's hope it never comes to that!

The mind can find no rest there. If a mind is safe because it is defective, if it cannot be brave without being angry, diligent without being greedy, quiet without being fearful, then it should be shaken and tossed out in a storm. You will live in such a dictatorship if you become the slave of a passion. Aren't you ashamed to put vices as the guardian of virtue?

Reason does not need the help of passion

If reason can do nothing without passion, then reason loses its power. It begins to be equal to passion and becomes like one. How are they different if passion without reason is as reckless as reason without passion is helpless? They are both on the same level if one cannot exist without the other. Yet who could tolerate that passion should be made equal to reason?

"Then," says our challenger, "passion is useful, provided it be moderate."

No, only if it is useful by nature. If it is disobedient to authority and reason, all we gain by its moderation is that the less there is of it, the less harm it does. Therefore, a moderate passion is nothing but a mild evil.

Think about this

If reason can do nothing without passion, then reason loses its power.

CHAPTER 11

Anger is Self-destructive

Key points of this chapter

1. *We don't have to be angry with our enemies. We can achieve our goal without being angry.*
2. *Anger destroys everything that comes its way. It is also self-destructive.*
3. *Virtue is controlled and not self-destructive. It brings itself to the front deliberately.*

Should we be angry with our enemies?

"But," argues our challenger, "against our enemies anger is necessary."

In no case is it less necessary. Our attacks should not be unruly but be measured and controlled. What is it except anger, so damaging to itself, that overthrows barbarians? This is despite their having so much greater bodily strength and the ability to endure fatigue better than us.

Gladiators also protect themselves by skill but expose themselves to harm when they are angry. Besides, what is the use of anger, if we can achieve the same result through the use of reason?

Do you think that a hunter is angry with the animals he kills? Yet he meets them when they attack him and follows them when they flee from him. All these are achieved by reason without anger.

Anger destroys

When thousands of Cimbri and Teutones poured over the Alps, they perished utterly. No messenger, only common rumor, carried the news of that great defeat to their homes.

What caused their collapse except that they were angry rather than courageous?

Anger destroys everything including itself

Anger sometimes overthrows and breaks to pieces whatever it meets. Yet more often it causes its own destruction.

Who can be braver than the Germans? Who can charge more boldly? Who has more love of arms among which they were born and bred, and only cared for them while neglecting everything else? Who can be more hardened to undergo every hardship, since most of them have no clothes to cover their body or shelter to protect them from the rigorous climate?

Yet Spaniards and Gauls, and even the unwarlike races of Asia and Syria, cut them down before the main legion comes within sight. Nothing but their own quick temper exposed them to death.

Give but intelligence to their minds and give but discipline to their bodies. They are now ignorant of vicious refinements, luxury, and wealth.

To say nothing more, we should go back to the ancient Roman habits of life.

- How did Fabius restore the shattered forces of the state, except by knowing how to delay, which angry people cannot do? The empire, then at its last gasp, would have perished if Fabius had been as daring as anger nudged him to be. But he thought about the conditions. After counting his force, he realized that he could lose no part of it without losing everything else with it. He set aside thoughts of grief and revenge and focused his attention on the best course of action to make the most of his opportunities. Thus, he conquered his anger before he conquered Hannibal.
- What did Scipio do? Did he not leave behind Hannibal and the Carthaginian army, and everyone with whom he had a right to be angry? Did he not carry over the war into Africa so deliberately that he made his enemies think he was luxurious and lazy?
- What did the second Scipio do? Did he not remain a long, long time before Numantia? Did he not calmly bear the criticism directed at him and his country that Numantia took longer to conquer than Carthage? By blocking his enemies, he brought them to such straits that they killed themselves.

Virtue does not harm itself

Anger, therefore, is not useful even in wars or battles, because it tends to be reckless. While trying to bring others into danger, it opens itself to danger. The most trustworthy virtue considers itself long and carefully, controls itself, and slowly and deliberately brings itself to the front.

Think about this

Anger sometimes overthrows and breaks to pieces whatever it meets. Yet more often it causes its own destruction.

CHAPTER 12

Anger is Poison

Key points of this chapter

1. *If we need to avenge an injustice, it is possible to do it without being angry.*
2. *People get angry over trivial things. Yet they consider their anger to be righteous and therefore justified.*
3. *Anger is never useful, even if it appears beneficial sometimes.*

Can we avenge without anger?

"What, then," says our challenger, "should a good person not be angry if he sees his father murdered or his mother raped?"

No, he won't be angry, but he will avenge them or protect them. Why are you afraid that duty alone, without anger, will not motivate him? You may as well say,

"What then? When a good man sees his father or his son killed, I suppose he will not weep or faint," as we see women do whenever they hear any trivial rumor of danger.

The good person will do the duty of a good human being without distraction or fear and in such a way that it is not unworthy of a human being.

My father is going to be killed; then, I will defend him. He is killed; then, I will avenge him. Not because I am grieving, but because it is my duty.

Everyone considers their anger 'righteous'

To believe "Good people are made angry by injuries done to their friends" (Theophrastus) is to discredit stronger principles, leaving the judgment to the mob rather than to a judge.

Everyone is angry when such things happen to their friends. You think they can believe that it is for them to decide what they do. As a rule, everyone considers their anger as righteous.

But they do the same thing if the hot water is not ready for them to drink, if a glass is broken, or their shoe is splashed with mud. Anger is a sign of a weak mind, not of one driven by duty. It is like children crying, whether they lose their parents or lose their toys. To get angry on behalf of one's friends is not the sign of a loving mind, but a weak one.

It is admirable and worthy to defend one's parents, children, friends, and countrymen, when duty calls—not impulsively or furiously—but willingly, with deliberate judgment and foresight.

Anger is never useful

No emotion is more eager for revenge than anger, and, for that very reason, one should avoid it. Anger is unduly hasty and frantic. Like almost all desires, it blocks its own path. Therefore, it has never been useful either in peace or war. It makes peace like war, and when bearing arms, forgets that Mars belongs to neither side. Being powerless itself, it succumbs to the power of the enemy.

Anger is harmful, even if it is occasionally beneficial

Next, vices should not be brought into everyday use because, on some occasions, they have been somewhat effective. Even fevers are useful for certain kinds of ill-health, and yet it is better to be altogether free of them. It is a terrible cure to one's disease.

Anger, like poison, or falling headfirst, or being shipwrecked, may have unexpectedly positive consequences. Yet it should not, for that reason, be considered healthy. After all, even some poisons are beneficial for health.

Think about this

No emotion is more eager for revenge than anger. For that very reason, one should avoid it.

CHAPTER 13

Weakness Causes Anger

Key points of this chapter

1. *Anger is not good because more of it is not better.*
2. *Anger does not help people to be courageous. No vice can promote virtue.*
3. *An angry person is a weak person.*

Anger is not good, because more of it is not better

Desirable qualities become more desirable when we have more of them. If justice is a good thing, no one would say it is better to get rid of some part of it. If courage is a good thing, no one likes to diminish it in any way.

But, because it is not advisable to increase anger, it shouldn't exist at all. If it grows worse when increased, it cannot be a good thing.

Anger does not help courage

"Anger is useful," says our challenger, "because it makes men more ready to fight."

According to that line of reasoning, then, drunkenness is also is a good thing, because it makes men rash and daring. They use their weapons better when they are made worse by drinking.

Again, according to that reasoning, you can also call frenzy and madness essential to strength because madness often makes people stronger.

By contrary rules, doesn't fear make people bolder, and doesn't the terror of death provoke even total cowards to join the war?

Yet anger, drunkenness, fear, and the like, are despicable and temporary provocations to action. They cannot arm virtue, which does not need vices.

They may at times, however, be of some little help to lazy and cowardly minds. No one becomes braver through anger, except one who, without anger, would not have been brave at all. Anger does not, therefore, come to assist courage but to take its place.

An irritable person is a weak person

What are we to say to the argument that, if anger were a good thing, it would attach itself to all the best men? Yet the most irritable of creatures are infants, older adults, and sick people. Every weak person is naturally prone to complaining.

Think about this

Because it is not advisable to increase anger, it shouldn't exist at all. If it grows worse when increased, it cannot be a good thing.

CHAPTER 14

Don't be Angry at Offenders

Key points of this chapter

1. *It is not proper for a sensible person to be angry at a person who makes a mistake because we all make them.*
2. *The kind thing to do is to gently correct their mistake rather than to be angry at them.*

Theophrastus says that it is impossible for good people not to be angry with bad people. By this reasoning, the better a person is, the more irritable she will be. Would she not rather be more tranquil, free from passions, and hating no one? What reason does she have for hating wrongdoers, since it is error that leads them into such crimes?

A sensible person doesn't hate those who err

It is not proper for a sensible person to hate those who err because it is like hating oneself. Let reasonable people think how many things they do contrary to good morals, how much of what they have done needs pardoning. Then they will soon become angry with themselves too.

No righteous judge pronounces a different judgment in their own case than in that of others. We cannot find anyone who can acquit himself. Everyone who calls himself innocent looks to external witnesses rather than to his own conscience.

How much kinder it is to deal with the those who err in a gentle and paternal way, and to direct them to the right course than to punish them. When someone wanders about our fields because they have lost their way, it is better to place them on the right path than to chase them away.

Think about this

How much kinder it is to deal with the those who err in a gentle and paternal way and to direct them to the right course than to punish them.

CHAPTER 15

Anger and Punishment Don't Mix

Key points of this chapter

1. *Punishment is a form of correction and should not arise out of anger.*
2. *Punishment may be dreadful, but sometimes it may be the only cure.*
3. *Punishment should never be carried out in anger*

Punishment should not arise out of anger

Therefore, the offender should be corrected both by warning and by force, both by gentle and harsh means. Thus, they may be made better people both towards themselves and others, But by reprimand, not anger. Who would be angry with the patient while nursing their wounds?

Punishment as correction

"But they cannot be corrected, and there is nothing in them that is gentle or hopeful."

If they are likely to corrupt everyone they meet, then let us remove them from the society of the living. Let them cease being bad in the only way they can. Let's do this without hating the person. What reason do we have for hating the person to whom we are doing the highest good and rescuing them from themselves? Do we hate our limbs when we need to cut them off? It is not an act of anger but a regrettable method of healing.

Punishment as a dreadful cure

We knock rabid dogs on the head, and we kill ferocious bulls. We doom scabby sheep to the knife, so they don't infect the flock. These are not acts of anger, but dreadful methods of healing.

We destroy monstrous births. We also drown our children if they are born weak or unnaturally formed. To separate what is useless from what is sound is not an act of anger, but an act of reason.

Punishment and anger don't go together

A penalty is more potent if it is carried out without rage. Therefore, nothing is less suitable than for the punisher to inflict the punishment with anger.

When punishment is the result of deliberate judgment, it has the power to reform. This is why Socrates said to the slave, "I would strike you, were I not angry." He put off punishing the slave to a time when he would not be angry. For now, he corrected himself.

Who can boast that they have their passions under control when Socrates did not dare to trust himself to his anger?

Think about this

"I would strike you, were I not angry."—Attributed to Socrates.

CHAPTER 16

The Wise Do Not Punish in Anger

Key points of this chapter

1. *The wise do not punish others because they are angry. They punish to correct the offender.*
2. *There are different kinds of punishments, depending on the nature and severity of the offense.*
3. *The wise will hand out the right sentence but will not be angry with the offender.*
4. *The wise may feel mildly emotional about it, but not much.*

The wise punish to correct the offender

So, we don't have to be angry punishers to punish the offenders and the depraved. Anger is a crime of the mind. It is not right to punish one offense with another.

There are different levels of punishment

"What! Shouldn't I be angry with a thief, or a poisoner?"

No. It's like my not getting angry with myself when I bleed. [Depending on the context], I apply different kinds of punishment as remedies:

- Now you are only in the first stage of error. You have not gone wrong seriously, although your lapses are frequent. I will try to correct you by warning in private and then in public.
- Now you have gone too far to be brought back to virtue by words alone. You must be kept in order by shame.
- For the next level, some more robust measure is required, something that marks you as the offender. You, sir, shall be sent into exile and to a deserted place.
- The next person's extensive crimes need harsher remedies: restraints and prison.
- You, lastly, have an incurably vicious mind, and add crime to crime. You have gone so far that you are not influenced by the arguments that don't include evil. To you, sin itself is a sufficient reason for sinning. Your whole heart is so soaked in evil, that evil cannot be taken from you without bringing your heart with it. Miserable man! You have wanted to die for so long. We will help you. We will take away your madness from which you suffer. You who have so long-lived a misery to yourself and to others, we will give the only good thing which remains, that is, death.

Why should I be angry with a man just when I am doing him good? Sometimes the sincerest form of compassion is to put a man to death.

Punishments depend on the offense

If I were a skilled and learned physician and entered a hospital or a rich person's house, I would not prescribe the same treatment for all patients; they may have different diseases.

I see different kinds of vice in different minds, and I am asked to heal the whole body of citizens.

Let us look for the proper remedy for each disease. This man may be cured by his own sense of honor, that one by travel, that one by pain, that one by need, that one by the sword.

Suppose it becomes my duty as a magistrate to put on black robes and summon an assembly by the sound of a trumpet. I won't walk to the seat of judgment with anger or hostility, but with the attitude of a judge. I will pass the formal sentence in a serious and gentle rather than an angry voice. I will ask them to proceed firmly but not angrily.

Even when I order a criminal to be executed, when I require someone to be punished for the murder of a close relative, when I order another to be punished under military law, or when I order a traitor to be thrown down the Tarpeian Rock, I will not be angry. I will look and feel as I do when I'm crushing snakes and other poisonous creatures.

The law is not outraged at the offender

"Anger is necessary to enable us to punish."

Really? Do you think that the law is angry with people it does not know, whom it has never seen, whom it hopes would never exist? We should, therefore, adopt the law's frame of mind, which does not become angry, but merely defines offenses.

If it is right for a good person to be mad at serious crimes, it will also be right for that person to be envious of the prosperity of the criminal.

What is more shocking than that, in some cases, the people for whom no misfortune is bad enough flourish and become successful? Yet they will see their affluence without envy, just as they see the offender's crimes without anger.

A good judge condemns unlawful acts but does not hate the offender.

The wise may experience some emotion, not much

"What then? When the wise is dealing with something of this kind, will his mind not be affected by it and become excited beyond what is normal?"

I admit that it will. They will experience a slight and minor emotion. As Zeno says, "Even in the mind of the wise, a scar remains after the wound is quite healed."

They will, therefore, feel specific hints and traces of passions, but they will be free from the passions themselves.

Think about this

If it is right for a good person to be angry at serious crimes, it will also be right for that person to be moved with envy at the prosperity of the criminal.

CHAPTER 17

Anger is Inconsistent

Key points of this chapter

1. *We cannot use anger because anger has a life of its own, and we cannot bring it under our control.*
2. *Reason by itself is capable of taking care of us.*
3. *Reason is firm, and anger is not. Reason is consistent, and anger is not.*
4. *Reason is enough for us. We don't need the help of anger.*

Anger has a life of its own

Aristotle says that "certain passions if one makes proper use of them, act as arms."

This would be true if, like weapons of war, we could pick them up or put them down as we pleased. But these arms, which Aristotle considers to be a virtuous fight of their own accord, do not wait to be seized by the hand. They own us instead of being owned by us.

Reason by itself can take care of us

We don't need external weapons. Nature has trained us sufficiently by giving us a reason. It has given us a weapon that is strong and durable. It is under our control, and we can be sure it cannot be turned against us

Reason by itself is enough— not just to take care of the future, but to manage our affairs as well. What can be more foolish than for reason to beg anger for protection? Will what is certain beg of what is uncertain? What is trustworthy of what is faithless? What is well of what is ill? What, indeed?

Reason is far more potent by itself, even in performing tasks for which anger may seem helpful. Therefore, when reason decides that something should be done, it continues doing it, because it cannot find anything better than itself to deal with.

Reason is firm. Anger isn't

Reason, therefore, stands by its purpose once it is formulated. On the other hand, pity often overcomes anger because it possesses no firm strength. It merely puffs up like an empty bladder. It makes a violent beginning, just like the winds caused by rivers and marshes. They rise from the earth and blow furiously without any maintenance.

Anger begins as a powerful blast but gets tired too soon and loses steam. It thinks of nothing but cruelty and novel forms of torture, and yet it gets weak and mild when it is time to punish. Passion soon cools, but reason is always consistent.

Even when anger continues to burn, after the death of two or three, it stops slaying when many may deserve to die.

Anger is inconsistent

Anger starts aggressively, like snakes when aroused from their den. Their teeth are venomous at first but become harmless when repeated bites exhaust their poison. As a result, those who are equally guilty are not similarly punished. Often those who have done less are punished more because they fell in the way of anger when it was fresher.

It is totally inconsistent. At one time, it runs into undue excess; at another, it falls short of what needs to be done. It indulges its own feelings and gives sentence according to its quirks. It will not listen to evidence, will not let the defense present its case, and will do what it has wrongly assumed. Even when it is a mistake, it will not tolerate its opinion snatched from it.

Think about this

Anger starts aggressively, like snakes when aroused from their den. Their teeth are venomous at first but become harmless when repeated bites exhaust their poison.

CHAPTER 18

Anger Doesn't Listen

Key points of this chapter

1. *Reason listens to both sides of a story. Anger doesn't.*
2. *Reason is just. Anger just wants to be thought of as just.*
3. *Anger mistakes harshness for consistency.*

Reason listens, anger doesn't

Reason allows each side time to make its case. When more time is needed to discover the truth, reason demands it.

But anger is in a hurry. Reason wants to give a just decision; anger wants its verdict to be seen as just. Reason only looks at the matter in hand; anger is excited by irrelevant and peripheral things, unrelated to the case.

Anger is irritated by anything that comes close to a confident appearance, a loud voice, free speech, elegant clothing, high-sounding arguments, or popularity with the public. It often condemns a person because it dislikes their patron. It loves and maintains error even when the truth is staring it in the face. It hates to be proved wrong and thinks it is more honorable to persevere in its mistaken behavior than to retract it.

The story of Gnaeus Piso's anger

I remember Gnaeus Piso, who was free from many vices, and yet of a perverse temperament. He mistook harshness for consistency. In his anger, he ordered a soldier to be executed because he had returned from leave without his comrade. Piso had assumed that the soldier must have murdered his comrade if he could not show him. When the soldier asked for time for a search, Piso refused.

The condemned man was brought outside the rampart. When he was about to be executed, suddenly, his comrade, who was thought to have been killed, showed up.

So, the centurion in charge of the execution asked the executioner to lay down his sword, and led the condemned man back to Piso, to declare him innocent as events proved so. They were brought to the presence of their fellow soldiers. Everyone in the camp was happy and embraced one another. A big crowd accompanied them.

Piso angrily convened the tribunal and ordered them both to be executed. Neither of them murdered or was murdered.

What could be worse than this? Because one was proved to be innocent, two died. Piso even added a third: for he actually ordered the centurion, who had brought back the condemned man, to be executed as well. Three men were set up to die in the same place because one was innocent.

Anger invents reasons for its frenzy

O, how clever is anger at developing reasons for its frenzy!

"I order you to be executed," it says, "because you have been condemned to death; you, because you have been the cause of your comrade's condemnation; and you, because when I ordered you to put him to death, you disobeyed your general."

He discovered the means of charging them with three crimes because he could find no offense in them.

Think about this

Reason wants to give a just decision; anger wants its verdict to be seen as just.

CHAPTER 19

Anger vs. Rational Action

Key points of this chapter

1. *Anger is loud and agitated. Rationality is calm.*
2. *Anger is violent by nature. Rationality is not.*
3. *To hand out the appropriate punishment for offenses committed, one should be free of anger. Anger is not suited for this purpose.*

The difference between anger and reason

Irritability has this fault—it hates being ruled. It is angry with the truth itself if it comes against its will. It berates anyone it considers as its victim. It shouts and gestures with its entire body, together with criticisms and curses.

Reason does not act this way. But, if it becomes necessary, it silently and quietly wipes out whole households, destroys entire families of enemies of the state, demolishes their homes, and levels them to the ground.

It erases the names of those who are the enemies of liberty. It does all this without gnashing its teeth or shaking its head, or doing anything unbecoming of a judge, whose appearance should be particularly calm and composed at the time when she is pronouncing a critical sentence.

The violent nature of anger

Hieronymus asks, "Why do you have to bite your lips when you want to hit someone?"

What would he have said, had he seen a governor climb down from the court bench, snatch the wooden rod from the magistrate, and tear his clothes because those of others were not torn fast enough?

Why do you need to upset the table, throw drinking cups, knock yourself against the columns, tear your hair, beat your thigh, and your breast?

How violent must the anger be if it turns back upon itself because it cannot find someone else as the target? Such people, therefore, are held back by others who beg them to calm down.

The calm nature of rationality

But, if an anger-free person assigns a penalty to those that deserve it, none of this happens.

An anger-free person will often let people go who have committed an offense if they are remorseful, their criminality is only skin deep but not deep-rooted, and they are likely to behave better in the future. She will grant immunity to those whose offense will hurt neither them nor those on the receiving end.

An anger-free person deliberates

In some cases, she will punish severe crimes more leniently than less severe ones, if the former is the result of a momentary lapse, not of cruelty, and, the latter is the result of deceitful, underhanded, habitual deviousness.

The same offense committed by two separate people will not be given equal penalties if one was the result of carelessness, and the other was planned and intentional.

She will remember that one form of punishment is to make bad people better, and the other to put them away. In either case, she will look to the future, not to the past.

As Plato says, "no wise person punishes anyone because they have sinned, but that they may sin no more: for what is past cannot be recalled, but what is to come may be checked."

When she wants to show that crime doesn't pay, she executes the criminals publicly, so they may, by dying, deter others from committing crimes.

To punish, one should be free from anger

To evaluate and consider all this, a person should be free from mental disturbance because they are dealing with something that should be handled very carefully. This is a matter of life and death. The sword of justice is in the wrong hands with an angry person.

Think about this

The sword of justice is in the wrong hands with an angry person.

CHAPTER 20

Anger is Not Noble

Key points of this chapter

1. *Anger does not contribute to greatness.*
2. *A noble mind is different from a proud mind.*
3. *A mind cannot be noble if it is not good. An angry mind is not good; therefore, it is not noble.*

Anger does not contribute to greatness

We should not believe that anger contributes anything to greatness either. It is not greatness but narcissism. It is like a disease that causes bodies to swell with unhealthy fluids. It is not growth but a bloating of the body.

Those whose insanity is above human consideration believe that great and sublime ideas inspire them. But they have no ground to stand on, and what is without foundation will likely collapse and slide into ruin.

Anger has no ground to stand on, and it is not built on a firm and steady foundation. It has a fleeting and empty quality, which is as far removed from greatness as recklessness is from courage, conceit from confidence, scarcity from simplicity, and cruelty from discipline.

The difference between a noble and a proud mind

There is a big difference between a noble and a proud mind. Anger doesn't bring about anything tremendous or beautiful. It seems to me that, to be always be irritated is the result of a lazy and unhappy mind, conscious of its own weakness. It is like those with sick bodies covered with sores and hurt at the slightest touch.

Anger, therefore, is a vice which, for the most part, affects women and children. Yet it affects men also. Because many men, too, are womanish or have the intellectual capacity of a child.

"But what can we say? Don't some angry words appear to flow from a great mind?"

Yes, to those who don't know what true greatness is. For example, I am sure that the offensive and hateful saying, "Let them hate me, provided they fear me," was written in Sulla's time. I don't know what thought was worse—being hated or feared. He thought that someday people would curse him, plot against him, crush him.

What prayer does he add to this? May all the gods curse him for discovering a cure for hate so worthy of it. "Let them hate." How?

"Provided they obey me?"

No!

"Provided they approve of me?"

No!

"How then? "

"Provided they fear me!"

I don't even want to be loved under that condition. Do you imagine that this was supposed to be high spirited? Wrong! This is not greatness but a monstrosity. You should not believe the words of the angry whose speech is very loud and threatening, but their minds are as timid as can be.

One has to be good to be great

Don't suppose either that the most eloquent of men Titus Livius was right in describing somebody as being "of a great rather than a good disposition." They cannot be separated.

One must be good to be great, because a great mind is unshaken, always sound, and its foundation is firm and uniform. It cannot exist along with evil nature, which is terrible, frantic, and destructive. Such qualities cannot possess greatness because greatness rests upon goodness and draws its strength from it.

"Yet by speech, action, and all outward show, they will make others believe that they are great."

True, they will say something, and you may think it shows a great spirit. For example, Gaius Caesar was angry with heaven because it interfered with his ballet dancers. He imitated them carefully rather than paying attention to them when they performed. Because Jupiter frustrated his enjoyment by his thunders, he challenged him to fight to the death, shouting the Homeric verse:

Carry me off, or I will carry thee!

How great was his madness! He either believed that he could not be hurt even by Jupiter, or that he could hurt Jupiter himself.

I imagine that his challenge encouraged the conspirators. It might very well have been the height of their endurance to tolerate someone who could not tolerate Jupiter.

Think about this

You should not believe the words of the angry, whose speech is very loud and threatening, but their minds are as timid as can be.

CHAPTER 21

Anger is Confused

Key points of this chapter

1. *There is nothing grand or noble in anger.*
2. *Angry people assume that extravagance, greed, lust, and ambition produce greatness.*
3. *Nothing is great unless it is also peaceful at the same time.*

Nothing is great if it not peaceful at the same time

Therefore, there is nothing exceptional or noble in anger, not even when it seems to be powerful or scornful of both gods and humans.

- Anyone who thinks that anger produces greatness would also believe that extravagance creates greatness. Such a person would wish to rest on ivory, dressed in purple, covered in gold, to move lands, dam seas, to hurry rivers, build forests in the air.

- He would think that greed shows greatness of mind because he clutches piles of gold and silver, treats the entire province as his estate, and owns large estates that extend beyond what was assigned to him under single bailiffs.
- He would think that lust shows greatness of mind. The lustful swim across straits, castrate crowds of boys, and make themselves open to the swords of injured husbands, and give no thought to death.
- He would think ambition, too, shows greatness of mind. The ambitious are not content with office once a year. If possible, they would fill the calendar of dignities with their name alone and cover the whole world with their titles.

It doesn't matter how far passions may go. They are narrow, pathetic, groveling. Virtue alone is lofty and sublime. Nothing is great unless it is also peaceful at the same time.

Think about this

Nothing is great unless it is also peaceful at the same time.

SENECA'S "ON ANGER." BOOK 2

ANGER, AN IMPULSE OR A CHOICE?

CHAPTER 1

Anger is a Deliberate Choice

Key points of this chapter

1. *The question that needs answering is whether anger is the result of an impulse or a decision with our consent.*
2. *Impulses are simple. But anger is complex. Therefore, it needs our mind's permission.*

Is Anger impulsive or deliberate?

Novatus, in my first book, I dealt with a rich subject: vices are on a slippery slope, rolling downhill. We should now investigate more severe matters.

Is anger a deliberate choice or is it is an impulse? Do we voluntarily set it in motion, or, like many other passions, does it creep up without our being aware of it?

We should first explore these things so we may be able to handle weightier matters later. It is like bones, ligaments, and joints in our body—not pleasing to look at, and yet they provide the foundations for our body and are essential to its wellbeing. Next come the parts that give our features their beauty. After these comes color, which above all attracts the eye of the onlooker, completing the rest of the body.

Anger is a deliberate choice

It is beyond doubt that anger is stirred when it appears to us we have been injured. But the question is,

Did the anger follow directly from the appearance of the injury without any help from our mind, or was it provoked with the help of the mind?

We [the Stoics] hold that anger does not start by itself without the mind's approval, because:

- to conceive the idea that a wrong has been done;
- to decide to avenge it; and
- to combine the above two and conclude that we should have been injured and we need to avenge it,

cannot be the result of a mere impulse that came about without our approval.

Anger is too complex to be impulsive

An impulse is a simple act. This is a complex one, composed of several parts. You understand something has happened; you become indignant, condemn it, and want to avenge it. All these things cannot come about without your mind agreeing to them.

Think about this

Impulse is a simple act. This [anger] is a complex one, composed of several parts. You understand something has happened; you become indignant, condemn it, and want to avenge it. All these things cannot come about without your mind agreeing to them.

CHAPTER 2

Anger and Involuntary Responses

Key points of this chapter

1. *Some of our emotional responses are involuntary. They cannot be considered as anger.*
2. *Anger is a defect of the mind and can be controlled.*
3. *We involuntarily respond to many things even when we are not directly involved. Such emotional responses are not passions but a prelude to them.*

Some of our reactions are involuntary

You ask, "What is the purpose of this inquiry?" We want to know what anger is.

If it comes about against our will, it will never be subject to reason. Anything that happens independent of our will is beyond our control and unavoidable—such as shivering when cold water is thrown over us, shrinking when we are touched in certain places, our hair standing on end at bad news, our faces blushing at obscene words, or getting dizzy when looking down a precipice.

It is not in our power to prevent any of these things. No reasoning can prevent their taking place.

Anger is a defect of the mind

But anger can be fought by rational principles, because it is a voluntary defect of the mind. It is not among those things that are the result of our human condition and happen even to the wisest of us. We should include in this list the initial mental jolt, which seizes us when we believe we have been wronged. We feel this way even when watching a play or reading about what happened a long time ago.

Sometimes we are not even directly involved

We often feel angry with Clodius for banishing Cicero, and with Antonius for murdering him. Who is not angry with the wars of Marius, the prohibitions of Sulla? Who is not furious at Theodotus and Achillas and the boy king who dared to commit an adult crime?

Sometimes songs excite us, as well as quickened rhythm and the noise of martial trumpets. Shocking pictures and the grim sight of punishments, however well deserved, affect our minds as well.

For the same reason, we smile when others smile, we are sad when we see a crowd of mourners, and we take a glowing interest in watching others compete. These feelings are not a different type of anger any more than what causes us to frown when we see a shipwreck is sadness. Neither is it fear that crosses our minds as we read of Hannibal's siege of Rome after Cannae.

A potential prelude to anger

All these are involuntary movements of minds. They are not passions, but seeds that may grow into passions. In the same way, a soldier is stirred at the sound of a trumpet even when he is in civilian clothes in peacetime, and the camp horses prick up their ears at the clatter of arms. They say that when Xenophantus was singing, Alexander's hand moved towards his sword.

Think about this

Anger can be fought by rational principles, because it is a voluntary defect of the mind.

CHAPTER 3

Anger Cannot Happen Without Our Assent

Key points of this chapter

1. *Our immediate impressions that are involuntary are not passions.*
2. *Involuntary actions subside unless we accept our impressions as real.*
3. *When we accept an impression of an injury as real, passions such as anger take us over.*

Body impulses are not passions

We should not call things that casually influence the mind "passions." The mind does not cause them but experiences them. So, passion does not mean that we are merely affected by the impressions we receive. Instead, it means that we give way to our emotions in response to these chance promptings.

Anyone who imagines that turning pale, bursting into tears, feeling lust, sighing deeply, sudden flashing of the eyes, and the like are signs of passion and reveal the state of mind, is mistaken and does not understand that these are merely impulses of the body. Thus, even the bravest often turn pale while they are putting on their arms.

- The knees of the most heroic soldiers shake a bit when they hear the battle signal.
- The heart of a great general leaps into his mouth before the opposing armies clash.
- The hands and feet, even of the most eloquent orators, grow stiff and cold while they are preparing to begin their speech.

Anger, a movement that's out of our control

Anger is not just a movement but, being impulsive, it breaks the bounds. This cannot happen without the consent of the mind. It is not possible to deal with revenge and punishment, without our mind knowing about it.

A person may think herself injured, may wish to avenge her wrongs. But then she may be persuaded by some reason or other to give up her intention and calm down. I do not call that anger, because it is a movement of the mind which is under the control of reason.

Anger cannot happen without our assent

Anger goes beyond logic and carries it away. Therefore, when struck, the first impression of an injury is no more anger than the impression itself. It is the mad rush that follows when one believes the impression of an apparent injury and acts upon it. Anger, the arousal of the mind to avenge, is a deliberate choice.

There can be no doubt that fear results in flight, and anger results in a pursuit. Consider, then, whether you think that anything can be either sought or avoided without the mind assenting to it.

Think about this

Passion does not mean that we are merely affected by the impressions we receive. Instead, it means that we give way to our emotions in response to these chance promptings.

CHAPTER 4

Involuntary Responses Are Not Passions

Key points of this chapter

1. *Our initial impressions are automatic.*
2. *We assent to the impression of injury and formulate a vengeful thought.*
3. *This assent we give the impression overrules reason.*

How anger begins and grows

Here is how passions start, grow, and gain momentum.

- The initial impression is involuntary. It prepares you for a passion, so to speak. It is a threatening signal.
- Next, it is combined with a desire—not a stubborn one, though—"I am injured, and so I should be avenged," or "This person should be punished for committing a crime."

- The third step is already beyond our control because it overrules reason and wants revenge, whether appropriate or not.

We cannot use reason to escape from that first impression on the mind, any more than we can escape the other involuntary movements of the body we talked about. We cannot prevent other people's yawns or cause ours; we cannot help closing our eyes when someone pokes their fingers at them.

Reason is unable to overcome these movements, even though they may perhaps be weakened by practice and constant vigilance. These are different from mental movements that are born of deliberation and can be ended by deliberation

---

Think about this

We cannot use reason to escape from that first impression on the mind, any more than we can escape the other involuntary movements of the body we talked about.

CHAPTER 5

Cruelty is Beyond Anger

Key points of this chapter

1. *Some people delight in hurting others, even though they received no injury.*
2. *People like that are not angry but possessed by an incurable disease.*

Anger vs. cruelty

Let's talk about those who are cruel, and who take pleasure in shedding human blood. Are they angry when they kill people who have done them no harm, and they themselves are aware of it? I mean the likes of Apollodorus or Phalaris.

This is not anger; it is ferocity. It is not retribution for an injury. It doesn't even mind being injured as long as it can harm. It doesn't seek to avenge when it kills but only to derive pleasure.

What can we say then? This evil starts from anger that has lost any thought of mercy and human connection by its frequent use. It finally becomes cruel.

Cruel people take delight in their cruelty

Such people smile with delight and enjoy themselves. They don't look angry like angry people do, because they find relaxation in their brutality. They say that when Hannibal saw a ditch full of human blood, he cried out, "What a beautiful sight!" How much more beautiful would he have found it if it had filled a river or a lake?

Why should we be surprised that, above all, he was mesmerized by this sight? After all, he was born in bloodshed and was brought up amid the slaughter from a child.

For twenty years, fortune will follow him, support his cruelty, and show him everywhere sights he loves—around Lake Trasimene, around Cannae, and finally around his city, Carthage.

Cruelty is an incurable disease

Not long ago, Volesus, the governor of Asia Minor under the Emperor Augustus, beheaded three hundred people. Then he strode about among the corpses with a superior look, as though he had done something grand and noble, exclaiming in Greek, "What a royal action!"

What would he have done if he had been a real king? This is not anger but a deeper and incurable disease.

Think about this

This evil [cruelty] starts from anger that has lost any thought of mercy and human connection by its frequent use. It finally becomes cruelty.

CHAPTER 6

Virtue is Not Angry at Vice

Key points of this chapter

1. *Virtue is not angry, because virtue and vice do not mix.*
2. *Violent and frequent anger doesn't belong to the wise.*

Should virtue be angry at what is mean?

"Virtue," argues our challenger, "should be angry with what is mean, just as it applauds what is honorable."

What would we say if he said that virtue should be both mean and magnificent? Yet this is what he means. He wants virtue to be raised up and debased.

Joy derived from a good action is grand and glorious, while anger at another's wrongdoing is mean and a sign of narrow-mindedness. Virtue will never make the mistake of imitating vice while seeking to control it.

Virtue holds that anger must be chastised since it often is even more criminal than the faults with which it is angry. Virtue is, by its very nature, joyful. It is as much beneath its dignity to be angry, as to grieve. Sorrow is the companion of anger, and all anger turns into sadness, either from remorse or from rebuff.

Again, if it is proper for the wise to be angry at wrongdoing, they will be angrier more often, the greater they are. It follows that the wise will not only be angry but quick-tempered.

Frequent anger doesn't belong to the wise

If we do not believe that great and frequent anger can find any place in the mind of the wise, why should we not set them altogether free from this passion? There can be no limit to anger if anger is proportional to what everyone does. They will either be unjust and equally angry at unequal crimes or be the quickest tempered of human beings if they fly into a rage as often as crimes merit their anger.

Think about this

If we do not believe that great and frequent anger can find any place in the mind of the wise, why should we not set them altogether free from this passion?

CHAPTER 7

Unworthy People Are Everywhere

Key points of this chapter

1. *The wise cannot be angry with the unworthy because there are too many unworthy people.*
2. *Therefore, if the wise get angry with the unworthy, they will be perpetually angry.*

The wise cannot be upset by the unworthy

What can be more unworthy of the wise, than that their passions depend upon the badness of others? If so, will the great Socrates ever be able to return home with the same expression he had when he left?

Besides, if it is the duty of the wise to be angry at shameful behavior, and to be upset and saddened at crimes, then no one is more unhappy than the wise. They will spend all their life in anger and grief.

Will there be an instant when they do not see something deserving of blame? Whenever they leave their house, they will be obliged to walk among criminals, misers, spendthrifts, and the shameless, who are happy in being who they are. The wise cannot cast their glance in any direction where they wouldn't see something to shock them. They will faint if they are angry as often as reason calls for it.

The world is full of unworthy people

Thousands of people are hurrying to go to the law courts at dawn. How shameful are their cases? How much more shameful are their advocates? One brings a lawsuit against his father's will when he would have done better not to deserve it. Another accuses his mother. A third comes to act as an informer against someone on a charge of which he is clearly guilty. A judge is chosen to condemn others for doing what he himself has done. The onlookers side with the guilty led astray by the delicate voice of the advocate.

Think about this

The wise cannot cast their glance in any direction where they wouldn't see something to shock them. They will faint if they are angry as often as reason calls for it.

CHAPTER 8

People vs. Wild Animals

Key points of this chapter

1. *There are as many vices as there are people.*
2. *People with vices behave like wild animals.*
3. *Yet, wild animals don't attack their keeper, but people do.*

There are as many vices as there are people

Why do I go through individual cases? When you see the court packed with a mob, the polling place swarming with people, or the circus where most people gather, be sure that there are as many vices among them as there are people.

People you see in civilian clothes are continually fighting among themselves. They will ruin each other for a small profit. No one profits except by someone else's loss. They hate the rich and despise the poor. They resent the great and harass the low. They are spurred by a host of desires and would destroy everything for the sake of a little pleasure or loot.

Animals don't attack their keepers, people do

They fight with the people they live with, as though they were in a gladiatorial school. It is like a society of wild animals, except that animals live peacefully among themselves. They don't bite their own, but these people tear one another and consume one another.

But there is one difference between them and dumb animals. Animals behave gently with their keepers, while the rage of people bites the very hand that feeds them.

Think about this

There is one difference between them and dumb animals. Animals behave gently with their keepers, while the rage of people bites the very hand that feeds them.

CHAPTER 9

The Wise and The Vicious

Key points of this chapter

1. *People commit a wide variety of crimes.*
2. *If the wise get upset about crimes, they will practically go insane.*

Once they begin, the wise will never be able to stop being angry because every place they come across is full of vices and crimes. More crimes are committed than can be healed by punishment. We seem to be engaged in a big struggle with wickedness.

People perpetrate a wide variety of crimes

Every day people are increasingly eager to do wrong with diminishing modesty. Consideration for what is better and just has been cast out. Lust rushes to wherever it thinks fit. Crimes are no longer committed in secret. They happen before our eyes. Wickedness has become so common and gained such power in everyone's mind that innocence, instead of being rare, ceased to exist altogether.

Are lawbreakers isolated individuals? Are they just a handful? No. Do they break laws one at a time or even a few at a time? No. They have arisen everywhere, as though they are responding to a signal to wipe out the difference between right and wrong.

- The host is not safe from the guest.
- Father-in-law is not safe from son-in-law.
- There's seldom any goodwill between brothers either.
- Wives want to destroy their husbands.
- Husbands want to kill their wives.
- Stepmothers grow deadly poisonous plants.
- Young heirs wonder when their benefactors will die.

The list of crimes is endless

These are only a small part of people's crimes! The list has not described one people divided into two hostile camps—parents and children enrolled on opposite sides, Rome set on fire by the hand of a Roman, aggressive horseback riders tracking the hiding places of the proscribed, poisoned wells, plagues created by humans, trenches dug by children to put parents under siege, crowded prisons, fires that consume whole cities, deadly tyrannies, secret plots to establish royal power and executions, and people glorifying acts which were counted as crimes—I mean rape, debauchery, and lust.

Add to these, public laws of national bad faith, broken treaties, the stronger taking everything that the weak cannot defend, cheating, theft, fraud, and disowning of debt—too many crimes for our three law-courts to handle.

If you want the wise to be angry as the crimes warrant, they would not just be angry but would go insane.

Think about this

Every day people are increasingly eager to do wrong with diminishing modesty. Consideration for what is better and just has been cast out.

CHAPTER 10

Wrongdoing is Widespread

Key points of this chapter

1. *We should not be angry at people's faults. It is natural for them.*
2. *Wrongdoing is widespread.*
3. *The wise will treat wrongdoers kindly to contain evil, not necessarily to eradicate it.*

We shouldn't be angry at people's faults

You'd better think about this: We shouldn't get mad at people's weaknesses. What can we say to someone who is angry at someone who stumbled in darkness? Or at a deaf person because he cannot hear their orders? Or at children, because immersed in their games and silly jokes, they forgot what they were asked to do? What if you choose to be angry with the infirm for being sick, for growing old, or becoming tired?

Our intellects are confused

Among humanity's misfortunes is this: Our intellects are disordered. They not only cannot help going wrong but love it too. To avoid being angry with people, you must forgive all at once. You should pardon the entire human race. If you are angry with the young and old because they do wrong, you will be angry with infants also, because they too will do wrong soon.

No one becomes angry with children who are too young to understand the difference. Yet, to be a human being is a bigger and a better excuse than to be a child.

We are born as humans, subject to many mental and physical disorders. We are neither dull nor slow, but we misuse our insight and our intellect. For example, we lead one another into vice by our example.

We can excuse anyone who follows others on the wrong road, for having wandered on the highway. A general may punish individual deserters severely. But when the whole army deserts, it must be pardoned.

Wrongdoing is widespread

What stops the wise person from being angry? It is the number of wrongdoers. The wise see how unjust and how dangerous it is to be angry with vices that everyone shares.

Heraclitus, whenever he left his house and saw such a mass of people around him living miserably—no, rather dying miserably—he would weep. He pitied all those who met him who were joyous and happy. He was gentle but too weak. He himself was one of those for whom he should have wept.

Democritus, by contrast, is said never to have appeared in public without a smile. He found it hard to take people's occupations seriously. What is there to be angry about? Everything moves us either to tears or to laughter.

There are very few wise people

The wise will not be angry with wrongdoers. Why not? Because they know that no one is born wise but becomes so. They know that very few turn out to be wise at any given time. They completely understand the human condition.

No sane man becomes angry with nature. What can we say if someone chooses to be surprised that fruit does not hang on shrubbery, or to wonder at bushes and thorns not being covered with some useful berry?

No one is angry when nature excuses a defect. Therefore, the wise, being tranquil, deal candidly with mistakes. They are not enemies of wrongdoers, but the wise will set them straight.

The wise will leave their house every day with this thought in mind: "I will meet many who are drunkards, lustful, ungrateful, greedy, and excited by ambition." He will see all these with kindness, as a doctor does his patients.

The wise will treat the wrongdoers kindly

When your ship leaks freely through its opened seams, do you become angry with the sailors or the vessel itself? No. Instead, you try to fix it. You shut out some water, bail out some water, close all the holes that you can see. By working consistently, you counter unseen gaps that let water into the hold. You don't relax your efforts because as much water as you pump out runs in again.

We are in a prolonged struggle against constant and prolific evils. Not to eradicate them, but merely to make sure they don't overwhelm us.

Think about this

We are in a prolonged struggle against constant and prolific evils. Not to eradicate them, but merely to make sure they don't overwhelm us.

CHAPTER 11

Don't Fear the Angry

Key points of this chapter

1. *Anger is not as strong as its threats would imply.*
2. *We should not use anger to frighten others.*
3. *Those who cause fear in others are despised.*
4. *Whatever causes fear is not free of fear itself. So, we should be afraid of angry people.*

Our challenger says, "Anger is useful, because it keeps you from being despised and because it frightens wrongdoers."

Anger is not as strong as its threats

First, if anger is as strong as its threats, it is hated because it arouses fear. It is more dangerous to be hated than to be despised.

But if fear lacks strength, it is much more open to contempt, and cannot avoid ridicule. What is flatter than anger when it huffs and puffs without purpose?

Anger, even when it frightens, is not desirable

Second, a thing is not attractive just because it is frightening. I would not want fear, which is a weapon of a wild animal, to be a weapon for the wise as well. We fear fever, gout, consuming ulcers. Is there any good in any of them because we fear them? Quite the opposite. They are all despised, disgusting, and base, for the very reason they induce fear in us.

So also, anger is hideous, and we should not be afraid of it. Yet many are scared of it, just as children are fearful of an ugly mask. How about the fact that anger always rebounds upon the angry? Or that peaceful people are not feared?

Here you may want to remember the verse of Laberius. When it was delivered on the stage during a civil war, it caught the attention of everyone as though it expressed the national feeling.

He must fear many, whom so many fear.

Whatever causes fear is itself afraid

Nature has proclaimed that whatever becomes great by creating fear in others is not free from fear itself. How disturbed lions are at the faintest noises! How excited those fiercest of animals become at strange shadows, voices, or smells! Whatever is a terror to others, is a terror for itself.

There is no reason, then, for any wise person to wish to be feared. You don't need to think that anger is terrific because it strikes terror since even the most despicable things like poisonous insects are feared.

'Scarer' is a line hung with feathers. It is so named because it scares a large herd of wild animals and steers them into traps. Foolish creatures are frightened by silly things. The movement of chariots and the sight of their wheels turning around drives lions back into their cage. Elephants are terrified at the cries of pigs.

So also, we fear anger just as children fear the dark, or wild animals fear red feathers. It has nothing stable or robust, but it affects feeble minds.

Think about this

Anger is hideous, and we should not be afraid of it.

CHAPTER 12

Nothing is Too Hard for the Mind

Key points of this chapter

1. *We are capable of eradicating anger.*
2. *The human mind is strong enough to accomplish anything it sets out to do.*

Our challenger says, "You must erase wickedness if you want to erase anger. But neither of these things can be done."

Is erasing anger impossible?

In the first place, it is possible to avoid being cold in the winter and hot in the summer? You can protect yourself against seasonal extremes by being in a location that provides protection, or by training your body to be tough so it feels neither heat nor cold.

In the second place, turn this saying around: You must erase anger from your mind before letting virtues in because virtues and vices cannot coexist. No one can be angry and good at the same time any more than one can be both sick and well at the same time.

Nothing is too complicated for the mind

"It is not possible," says our challenger, "to remove anger from the mind completely. Human nature does not allow it."

Yet there is nothing so hard and challenging that our mind cannot overcome it with regular practice. There are no passions so fierce and independent that they cannot be brought under control by discipline.

The mind can carry out the orders it gives itself. Some have succeeded in never smiling. Some have stayed away from wine, sexual intercourse, or even drink of all kinds. Some are satisfied with short hours of rest and kept up a tireless vigil. People have learned how to run up the thinnest slanting ropes, to carry heavy burdens, scarcely within the capabilities of human strength, or to dive to enormous depths and to remain under the sea without any chance to breathe.

There are a thousand other instances of persistence overcoming all obstacles. They prove that nothing is complicated when the mind has set itself to endure. People that I have just mentioned either were not rewarded or received a reward that wasn't worthy of their painstaking effort. What great thing do people gain by applying their intellect to tightrope walking? Or carrying a heavy load on their shoulders? Or not giving in to sleep? Or to reach the bottom of the sea?

Yet their patient labor makes all these things happen for no great reward. Would we not then summon the aid of patience, when such a prize as the unbroken calm of a happy life awaits us? How great a blessing is it to escape from anger, that chief of all evils, along with frenzy, ferocity, cruelty, and madness, and whatever accompanies them?

Think about this

There is nothing so hard and challenging that our mind cannot overcome it with regular practice.

CHAPTER 13

Anger is Curable

Key points of this chapter

1. *There is no reason for us to defend anger.*
2. *Anger is avoidable. It is easier than most people suppose.*

Anger cannot be defended

There is no reason for us to justify such a passion as this. We cannot excuse its excesses by saying that it is useful or unavoidable. What vice is without its defenders? Yet this is no reason why you should say that anger cannot be erased.

Our evils are curable

The evils from which we suffer are curable. We were born with a natural bias towards good, so nature itself will help us if we try to correct our lives. The path to virtue is not steep and rough, as some people think. The approach lies on level ground.

I am not here to peddle false stories. The road to happiness is easy. Just make a start with good luck and the excellent help of the gods themselves. It is much harder to do what you are doing. What is more restful than a peaceful mind, and what more troublesome than an angry one? What is more relaxed than mercy, and what is more taxing than cruelty?

Modesty has free time, while vice is always busy. In short, all virtues are easy to cultivate, while vices are priced high. We should get rid of anger. Even those who say that we should keep it under control admit this to some extent. Let us get free of it altogether. There is nothing to be gained by it. Without it, we can more quickly and more justly put an end to crime, punish the bad, and amend their lives. The wise will do their duty in all things without the help of any evil passion. They will have no use for things that need observing, so they don't go out of control.

Think about this

The evils from which we suffer are curable. We were born with a natural bias towards good, so nature itself will help us if we try to correct our lives.

CHAPTER 14

Don't Make Anger a Habit

Key points of this chapter

1. *Anger should never become a habit.*
2. *When anger arises, we must hold it down.*
3. *Use patience to hold down anger.*

Guard yourself against anger

Anger, then, must never become a habit with us. Sometimes we may pretend to be angry to stir the sluggish, just as we arouse horses that are slow to start with goads and firebrands. We must sometimes apply fear to those who are not impressed with reason. Yet to be angry is of no more use than to grieve or to be afraid.

When it arises, hold anger down

"Don't situations arise that provoke anger?"

Yes, they do. But then, as always, we should hold it down. It is not difficult to conquer our spirit. It is like the way the athletes who pay attention wholly to the basest parts of themselves can endure blows and pain so that they may drain the strength of the opponent.

They do not strike when anger prompts them, but only when the opportunity invites them. They say that Pyrrhus, the exceptional trainer of gymnastic contestants, regularly used to ask his students not to lose their temper because anger upsets their skill and looks only for a way to harm.

Reason often urges patience where anger urges revenge and, where we could have been free of our first misfortune, we expose ourselves to worse ones.

Some people have been exiled because they couldn't bear to hear a single word of insult. They bring upon themselves the yoke of slavery because they are too proud to give up even a tiny bit of their liberty.

Think about this

Anger must never become a habit with us.

CHAPTER 15

Good Nature Doesn't Preclude Vices

Key points of this chapter

1. *Naturally, substantial and daring people are more prone to anger. They need the training to tame it.*
2. *Good nature does not mean freedom from vices.*

Our challenger says, "So you may be sure that anger has something noble about it, look at the free nations, such as the Germans and Scythians. They are most prone to anger."

Why free nations have angry citizens

Yes. This is because naturally daring and substantial people are prone to anger before they are tamed by discipline. Some passions are born of nature—just as good land, even when wasted, has a vigorous undergrowth. Trees grow tall in this fertile soil. So also, naturally, bold characters tend to be irritable. Their hot and fiery nature has no mean or trivial qualities. But their energy is misdirected. It happens with all those who come to the front solely by their natural abilities. Their minds, unless brought under control, degenerate from a courageous temper into habits of rashness and reckless daring.

Good nature is not free from vices

"Aren't minor vices such as tenderness, love, and modesty linked with gentler minds?"

Yes, and therefore I can show that a pleasant disposition has its own faults. Even proven superior nature does not exclude vices. Besides, nations that are free because they are wild like lions or wolves, and cannot command any more than they can obey. The strength of their intellect is not civilized but fierce and uncontrollable.

Now, no one can rule unless they can also be ruled. That's why, for the most part, countries with a milder climate have had empires. Those who live near the frozen north have an uncivilized temper, "just on the model of their native skies," as the poet puts it.

Think about this

A pleasant disposition has its own faults. Even proven superior nature does not preclude vices.

CHAPTER 16

Reason Should Guide Us

Key points of this chapter

1. *We should use reason to guide our decisions and not imitate other animals.*
2. *The irritable people may appear straightforward, but they are only simple-minded.*

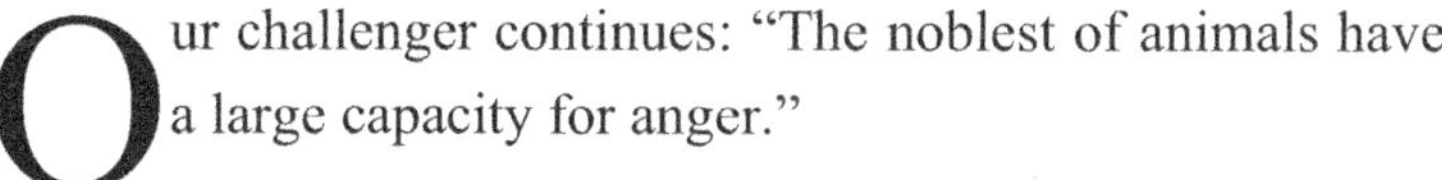

Our challenger continues: "The noblest of animals have a large capacity for anger."

Animals shouldn't be our models

It's a mistake to hold up impulsive animals rather than reason for humans to follow. Humans have reason in place of impulse.

Yet not even all animals are served by the same thing. Anger is of use to lions, timidity to deer, boldness to hawks, flight to doves. What if I say that it is not even true that the best animals are the most prone to anger? I suppose that predatory animals are better when they are angrier. However, I would praise oxen and horses for their patience when they obey the rein.

But why do you try to apply such poor models to human beings, when you have the universe and god, whom human beings alone comprehend?

The irritable people are heedless

"The most irritable people," says he, "are thought to be the most straightforward of all."

Yes, when compared to the deceitful and the tricky. They appear to be simple because they are outspoken. Yet, I would not call them straightforward, just heedless. We call all fools, gluttons, spendthrifts, and those whose vices lie on the surface "simple."

Think about this

It's a mistake to hold up impulsive animals rather than reason for humans to follow.

CHAPTER 17

Don't be a Robber or a Victim

Key points of this chapter

1. *Orators and actors are not angry but only pretend to be angry.*
2. *We should neither be too hard nor too soft. We should neither be a robber nor a victim.*

Our challenger says, "An orator is sometimes better when she is angry."

Orators just pretend to be angry

No, only when she pretends to be angry. Actors, too, move their audience though they are not angry when delivering the lines and acting angry. So it is when we are addressing a jury or a public forum or whenever we need to move the minds of others and influence them according to our will. We must pretend to be angry, fearful, or merciful ourselves before we can make others feel the same way. Often such acts achieve what genuine passions cannot.

One should be neither a robber nor a victim

"The mind which lacks anger is feeble," says our challenger.

True, if it has nothing stronger than anger to make it energetic. One should neither be a robber nor a victim, neither given to pity nor cruelty. The former belongs to a weak mind, the latter to a hard one. Let the wise be moderate, and when things call for courage, they should display strength, not anger.

Think about this

One should neither be a robber nor a victim, neither given to pity nor cruelty.

CHAPTER 18

Avoiding and Controlling Anger

Key points of this chapter

1. *We need strategies for avoiding anger as well as for controlling it once it has arisen.*
2. *Some of these strategies are specific to the young, and others are more general.*

Two types of prescriptions

We have so far discussed the questions concerning how anger arises. Let's now move on to its cures. As I see it, we have two objectives:

1. To stop becoming angry in the first place; and,
2. To prevent our doing wrong when angry.

Just as in taking care of our bodies where some prescriptions are for maintaining health and others for restoring it, we should both resist anger and control it once it has arisen.

Avoiding and controlling anger

For avoiding anger, I will offer some general rules which apply to all of us. I will divide this into two:

1. Rules that are useful during the education of the young; and,
2. Rules that are useful afterward.

Education calls for the greatest attention and will have the greatest payoff because it's easier to mold tender minds. It is difficult to uproot vices that we grow up with.

Think about this

Education calls for the greatest attention and will have the greatest payoff because it's easier to mold tender minds.

CHAPTER 19

The Four Elements and Our Disposition

Key points of this chapter

1. We *are a combination of four elements: fire, air, earth, and water.*
2. *Our dispositions incline to one or the other of these depending on the strength of each element in us.*

A passionate mind is, by nature, most vulnerable to anger.

There are four elements—fire, air, earth, and water—with four corresponding properties: hot, cold, dry, and moist. The blending of elements produces diverse lands and animals, bodies, and character. Our dispositions incline to one or the other of these depending on the strength of each element in us.

Hence it is that we call some areas wet or dry, warm or cold. The same distinctions apply to animals as well as to humans. It makes a significant difference in how much moisture or heat a person contains; their dominant element will shape their character.

A warm temper will make people more prone to anger because fire is full of movement and vigor. A mixture of coldness makes people cowards because cold is sluggish and constricted. Because of this, some Stoics think that anger is generated by the boiling of the blood around the heart. Indeed, that place is assigned to anger for no other reason than because the heart is the warmest part of the whole body. Those who have more moisture in them become angry slowly, because they have no heat ready at hand, and it has to be gained by movement. Therefore, the anger of women and children is sharp rather than stiff and arises on lighter provocation.

In dry times of life, anger is violent and powerful, but without an increase. It doesn't grow because heat dies, and cold takes its place.

Older adults are testy and full of complaints. So are the sick and the convalescent. Their reserve of heat has been used up by weariness or loss of blood. Those who are wasting away from thirst or hunger are in the same position, as are those who are naturally anemic and faint from starvation.

Wine kindles anger because it increases heat. According to each person's disposition, some fly into a passion when they are heavily drunk, some when they are slightly drunk. There is no other reason other than this why blondes and people with flushed complexions are prone to anger. They already have the color that others assume during anger. Their *blood is hot and quickly set in motion.*

Think about this

There are four elements: fire, air, earth, and water. Our dispositions incline to one or the other of these depending on the strength of each element in us.

CHAPTER 20

Mental Habits and Anger

Key points of this chapter

1. *Our dispositions can make us prone to anger.*
2. *Mental habits, however, have the greatest power. The right remedy will depend on things such as our disposition, and the type of anger we are trying to control.*

External causes of anger

Nature makes some people prone to anger. Many other factors have the same effect. Some have been led to this condition by disease or physical injury, others by hard work, sleeplessness, nights of anxiety, feelings of longing, and love. Anything that hurts the body or the mind stirs the disturbed mind to find fault. But these are only the first causes of anger.

The power of mental habits

However, mental habits have the greatest power. Unwholesome practices will nurture anger. We cannot change our nature; it was formed by the mixture of elements formed at our birth. Still, it will be useful to know that we should keep wine out of the reach of the passionate. (Plato thinks we should deny wine to children, so their fire doesn't grow fiercer.) We should not overfeed them because their body and mind will get bloated. They should exercise stopping short of fatigue so that they may lessen their natural heat. Games will also be useful.

Some remedies

Moderate pleasure relaxes the mind and brings it to a proper balance. Temperaments which incline to moisture, or dryness and cold, aren't at risk of anger. But they are subject to less spirited vices, such as cowardice, melancholy, despair, and suspiciousness. Therefore, their dispositions should be softened, comforted, and restored to cheerfulness.

Anger and despair call for different remedies. The remedies for two vices are not only different but diametrically opposed. Let us always attack the dominant one.

Think about this

The greatest power belongs to our mental habits. If they are unwholesome, they will nurture anger.

CHAPTER 21

Bringing up Children

Key points of this chapter

1. *Children derive the most significant benefit when you bring them up in a healthy way right from the start.*
2. *Bring children up in a way that supports their strengths but discourages their anger.*

Children benefit from right upbringing

I assure you, children derive the most significant benefit when you bring them up in a healthy way right from the start. Still, educating them is difficult because we need to avoid cherishing their anger without blunting their spirit. This requires careful monitoring. What we want to encourage and what we need to check look very similar and so can deceive us.

Bringing up children the right way

Children's spirit is fueled by freedom and dampened by control. It rises when praised and forms the right expectations. Yet, the same things can also produce anger and arrogance in a child. So, we should avoid extremes and guide them towards the middle path—sometimes by encouraging, sometimes by curbing.

- We should not subject children to anything degrading. Let them never beg for anything or gain anything by doing so. Let them get what they want for its own sake, for past good behavior, and future good quality conduct.
- Don't allow them to get sulky or angry when they are competing with their friends. Let's make sure that they are friendly with everyone they compete with, so they learn to win but not hurt others.
- When they win or do something worthy of praise, allow them to take delight in their success, but let them not swagger. Joy leads to jubilation, and jubilation leads to swaggering and excessive self-esteem.
- Allow them some relaxation, but don't allow them to be lazy or inactive.
- Keep them away from luxury. Nothing makes children more prone to anger than being brought up soft and spoiled. That's why the more we indulge an only child and give it more freedom, the more corrupt they become. Those who are not denied anything, whose anxious mother always wipes away their tears, whose attendant is made to pay for their faults, will not be able to withstand being offended. Don't you see how a person's anger

increases as their position rises? This is particularly true of the rich and the noble, with a favorable wind accompanying trivial and empty passions.

- Prosperity encourages anger. When a crowd of yes-men surrounds a proud person saying things like, "He talked back to you! If you do not act in line with your dignity, you lower yourself," and so on, even a principled and healthy mind will hardly be able to resist such language. So, we should keep children away from flattery. Let a child hear the truth and sometimes even fear it, but always have respect for it.
- Let them rise before their elders.
- Let them not gain any advantage by flying into a rage. Give them when they are calm what you refuse to give when they are angry, crying for it.
- Let them see, but not let them use, their father's wealth.
- Scold them when they do something wrong.
- It is helpful to give children teachers and attendants who are calm. What is tender and unformed clings to what is near and takes its shape. The young grow up to resemble those who nurtured and taught them. A boy who was brought up in Plato's house went home once to his parents and saw his father angrily shouting. He said, "I never saw anyone at Plato's house act like that." I don't doubt that he learned to imitate his father faster than he learned to imitate Plato.
- Above all, let their food be simple, their clothing inexpensive, and have them live the same way as their friends. If you begin by putting them on a level with many

others, they will not be angry when you compare someone with them.

Think about this

Children derive the most significant benefit when you bring them up in a healthy way right from the start.

CHAPTER 22

The First Cause of Anger

Key points of this chapter

1. *The first cause of anger is the perception that we are injured.*
2. *We should not immediately accept that we are injured because our perceptions can be wrong.*
    a. *Always give your anger some time.*
    b. *Don't listen to slanderous gossip.*
    c. *Guard yourself against hasty judgments.*

We discussed so far the rules that apply to our children. As far as we are concerned, we cannot fault or improve our accidental birth and our education. We can only deal with what follows.

The first cause of anger: perception of injury

Now we must fight against the primary causes of passion.

The cause of anger is the belief that we are injured. We should not casually accept this belief. We should not fly into a rage even when the injury appears to be clear and distinct, because some false things resemble truth.

Ways to deal with anger

- Always allow some time to elapse, for time reveals the truth.
- Do not listen to slanderous gossip.
- Know and be on your guard against this fault of human nature—we are willing to believe without wanting to listen, and we become angry before we have formed our opinion.

What can I say? We are influenced not just by slander but by suspicions. At the very look and smile of others, we may fly into a rage with innocent people because we interpret them in the worst possible way. We should, therefore, plead the case of those who are not present against ourselves. We need to suspend our anger. We can still inflict a postponed punishment but cannot recall an inflicted one.

Think about this

The cause of anger is the belief that we are injured. We should not casually accept this belief.

CHAPTER 23

Anger Can Turn on Well-wishers

Key points of this chapter

1. *Anger can turn on your well-wishers.*
2. *The best way to pardon people is not even wanting to know if they offended you.*

Anger destroys

Everyone knows the story of a tyrant who was captured before accomplishing his task of killing. Tortured by Hippias to name his accomplices, he named them while they were standing around, even though he knew that the tyrant's safety was important to them. As the tyrant ordered each man he named to be killed, he asked the last man if anyone else remained. The man replied, "You remain alone, for I have left no one else alive to whom you are dear."

Anger caused the tyrant to help Hippias to cut down his protectors with his own sword.

Alexander's moderation

How far more spirited was Alexander! His mother warned him to beware of poison from his physician, Philip. Alexander was undeterred and drank the medicine Philip gave him. He was more confident of his friend and was worthy of having a guiltless friend. I praise Alexander all the more for this because he was, more than anyone, prone to anger. The more uncommon moderation is among kings, the more it deserves to be praised.

Julius Caesar's mercy

The great Julius Caesar, who proved such a merciful conqueror in the civil war, did the same thing. He burned a packet of letters addressed to Gnaeus Pompeius by those who had been thought to be either neutrals or on the other side. Though Caesar was generally moderate in his anger, he nonetheless preferred not to be angry at all. He thought that the kindest way to pardon was not to know what the offense was at all.

Think about this

The more uncommon moderation is among kings, the more it deserves to be praised.

CHAPTER 24

Credulity Stokes Anger

Key points of this chapter

1. *Our credulity deceives us by uncritically accepting our impressions.*
2. *Our suspicion is cunning in finding 'proofs.'*
3. *What we need are directness and kindly judgment.*

Our beliefs lead us astray

Credulity makes the most mischief. Most of the time, you shouldn't even listen. In some matters, it's better to be deceived than to mistrust. You should totally get rid of suspicion and guesswork. They are the most unreliable goads to anger.

- That man greeted me with too little warmth.
- This woman broke off the kiss too quickly.
- That man quickly broke off a conversation I'd begun.
- This woman didn't invite me to dinner.

- That man had a slightly unfriendly look.

Suspicion will find the proof it needs

Doubt will discover evidence to support it. What we need are directness and kindly judgment. Let's believe nothing except what stares us in the face and is caught red-handed. Let's scold our credulity whenever our suspicion is empty. This sort of scolding will make us slow to believe as a matter of habit.

Think about this

What we need are directness and kindly judgment. Let's believe nothing except what stares us in the face and is caught red-handed. Let's scold our credulity whenever our suspicion is empty.

CHAPTER 25

Luxury Weakens the Mind

Key points of this chapter

1. *Petty things should not aggravate us.*
2. *Luxury weakens our body and mind.*
3. *We should train to toughen our minds.*

Don't be aggravated by petty things

From all the things we discussed, we can also see that we should not let petty and trivial things aggravate us. It is crazy to lose our temper because the servant is not quick, the water is lukewarm, the couch is disarranged, or our table carelessly set.

You must be in a miserably bad state of health if you shrink from a gentle breeze. Your eyes must be diseased if they are distressed by the sight of a bright white garment. You must be broken down by luxury if you feel pain seeing someone at work.

Luxury weakens the mind

They say that Mindyrides, a citizen of Sybaris, complained when he saw a man vigorously digging with his hoe that the sight made him tired and banned him from working from any place in his view. He also complained that he felt worse when he lay down on creased rose petals.

When pleasures have corrupted both the body and the mind, nothing seems bearable, not because it is hard, but because the person who has to bear it is soft.

Why should we be driven to frenzy by anyone's coughing and sneezing, or by a fly being chased without care, or by a dog's hanging about us, or a key dropping from a careless servant's hand?

If your ears are bruised by the noise of a bench being dragged along the floor, will you be able to bear calmly the abuses of public life, and the curses heaped on you in a public forum or the senate?

If you are angry with the waiter for icing your drink badly, will you be able to endure hunger and the thirst of a summer campaign?

We should train our mind to become tough

Nothing, therefore, feeds anger more than an excessive and dissatisfied luxury. We should toughen the mind by treating it rigorously, so it doesn't feel any blow that is not severe.

Think about this

Nothing, therefore, feeds anger more than an excessive and dissatisfied luxury.

CHAPTER 26

Avoid Irrational Anger

Key points of this chapter

1. *We get angry at inanimate objects as though they can harm us.*
2. *We also get angry with animals. Animals are not capable of forethought, so what they do is not intentional. Children and adults with reduced capacity belong to the same category.*
3. *We should distinguish injuries of ignorance from injuries of intention.*

We are angry either with those who can injure us or with those who cannot.

Anger at inanimate objects

Things that cannot injure us include inanimate objects, such as a book. We often throw it away if the print is too small for us to read or tear it up when it is full of mistakes. We destroy our clothes if we do not like them. How foolish to be angry with such things as these, which neither deserve nor feel our anger!

"But of course, it is those who make them that really offend us."

In the first place, we often become angry before making this distinction clear in our minds.

Secondly, maybe the publishers themselves have reasonable excuses. One of them could be that it was [technically] not possible to make it any better; no disrespect to you was intended.

Another reasonable excuse could be that they did what they did without having any intention of insulting you.

Finally, how absurd it is to vent out your spleen against things as if it is against people?

Anger at animals

It is as crazy to be angry with dumb animals as it is to be angry with inanimate objects. They can do you no wrong because they don't *intend* to injure you. We cannot call anything a wrong unless it is done intentionally. They are, therefore, able to hurt us, just as a sword or a stone may do, but they can do us no wrong.

Harm implies intent

Yet some people think themselves insulted when the horses that obey one rider defy another, as though it was their deliberate choice, and not because of habit or the rider's skill. It is foolish to be angry with them, as it is to be angry with children, and with people who have little more sense than children.

A fair judge would consider all these as ignorance. For a just judge, ignorance would be as effective a plea as innocence for such misdeeds.

Think about this

We cannot call anything a wrong unless it is done intentionally.

CHAPTER 27

Things Happen for Our Benefit

Key points of this chapter

1. *Things that appear to harm us actually happen for our benefit.*
2. *When we reflect on our way of life, we will realize that our punishments are light compared to what we deserve.*

Certain things cannot harm us

There are certain things that cannot harm us. They can only be beneficial—like the immortal gods, who neither wish to nor can harm us. Their nature is calm and gentle. They are no more likely to wrong others than to wrong themselves.

Foolish people blame nature

Foolish people who don't know the truth hold gods answerable for storms at sea, severe rain, and long winters.

The natural phenomena by which we suffer or profit are not aimed at us. It is not for our sake that the universe causes summer and winter to succeed one another. They have laws of their own, according to which their divine functions are performed. We think too much of ourselves when we imagine that we are worthy of causing such great stirrings.

Everything happens to our benefit

None of these things happen to harm us. No, it is quite the opposite—they all happen for our benefit. I've said that some things cannot harm us, and some things would not harm us. To the latter category belong good people in authority, good parents, teachers, and judges whose punishment is similar to a surgeon using her knife and fasting and all other things that cause pain for our benefit.

Reflect on your way of life

Suppose we are being punished. Let's not just think of what we suffer, but also of what we have done. Let's reflect on our way of life. Provided we want to tell ourselves the truth, we'll undoubtedly decide we got off lightly compared to what we deserved.

Think about this

The natural phenomena by which we suffer or profit are not aimed at us. It is not for our sake that the universe causes summer and winter to succeed one another. They have laws of their own.

CHAPTER 28

None of Us is Faultless

Key points of this chapter

1. *None of us is faultless. We are not even marginally innocent.*
2. *Wrongdoers are most vocal about other wrongdoers' offenses.*
3. *When you are tempted to be angry with others, remember how many times you were unfairly treated.*

If we want to be impartial judges of everything, we should first convince ourselves of this: None of us is faultless. This is the source of most of our indignation: "I'm without fault. I've done nothing wrong." In fact, you don't *admit* to having done anything wrong.

We resent it when we are rebuked either by reprimand or actual punishment. Yet, at this very moment, we are doing wrong by adding arrogance and defiance to our misdeeds.

Who is there that can say they have broken no laws? Even if there is such a person, what a skimpy innocence it is to be legally "not guilty"! How much further do the rules of duty extend! How many things which are not to be found in the law book are demanded by filial feeling, kindness, generosity, equity, and honor?

We are not even narrowly innocent

Yet, we cannot even fulfill the narrowest definition of innocence. We have done what was wrong. We have thought of what was wrong. We have hoped for what was wrong. And we have encouraged what was wrong. In some cases, we have remained innocent—only because we didn't succeed.

Treat offenders more fairly

With all this thought in mind, let's treat offenders more fairly. Let's assume that those who rebuke us are right. In any case, let us not be angry with ourselves (who will escape our anger, if we are angry even with our own selves?), and least of all with the gods. Whatever unpleasantness we suffer comes from the common laws we are all governed by. It is not the fault of the gods.

"But diseases and pains attack us."

Well, people who live in a madhouse must have some way of escaping from it. Someone speaks ill of you. Think. Have you not spoken ill of them? Think of the many others you have spoken ill of. Don't think that they have wronged you; they are just repaying what they had received.

Some act with good intentions, some under compulsion, some in ignorance. Let us believe that even those who acted intentionally did not do so just to harm us. Some might have thought that they were saying something witty. Or they did what they did not out of any spite against us, but because they couldn't succeed unless they got us out of the way.

Remember when you were unfairly treated

We are often offended by flattery even though we are praised. Yet, how often have we ourselves been unjustly suspected? How often have we appeared to have done something wrong although it is not so? How many people have we come to like after hating them at first?

We will be able to keep ourselves from becoming angry straightway if we silently say to ourselves when each offense is committed:

"I have done this very thing myself."

Where, however, will you find so impartial a judge? The same people who lust after everyone's wife and think that a woman belonging to someone else is a sufficient reason for adoring her, will not allow anyone else to look at their own wife.

No one expects as much faithfulness as a traitor. The perjurers take vengeance on those who break their word. Lawyers who bring false charges are outraged if an action is brought against them. Those who are careless about their own morality cannot endure seeing the same in others.

We don't see our own vices

We have other people's vices before our eyes, and our own behind our backs. Hence it happens that a father, who is worse than his son, blames the son for throwing lavish parties. Those who disapprove of the least sign of luxury in others set no bounds to it when it comes to them. The tyrants are angry with the murderer, and the impious punish thefts.

Most of us are not angry with sins but only with the sinner. We will be more moderate if we question ourselves; "Have we committed any crime like this one? Did we ever fall into this type of error? Is it in our interest to condemn this conduct?

Think about this

We have other people's vices before our eyes, and our own behind our backs.

CHAPTER 29

Delay is the Greatest Cure

Key points of this chapter

1. *Delay in the ultimate cure for anger.*
2. *We should not readily believe what others tell us.*
3. *People lie for different reasons. They have their own motives to do so.*
4. *We should listen to both sides of the story before jumping to conclusions.*

The ultimate cure for anger is delay

The ultimate cure for anger is delay. Ask anger not to pardon but to deliberate first so it may form a proper judgment about it. If it delays, it will come to an end. Don't attempt to quash it all at once, for its first impulses are intense. Pluck it away bit by bit, and you will remove it entirely.

Do not believe what you hear from others

Some things that make us angry, we learn from others. Other things we see or hear for ourselves. We shouldn't be quick to believe what others tell us.

Some people lie to deceive us, and others say things because they themselves are deceived. Some try to ingratiate themselves to us through false accusations and invent wrongs, so they may appear angry because others are unfair to us. One lies out of spite to split up a close friendship. Another is eager for some entertainment, watching from a safe distance the clash between the people she split up.

Do not judge before listening to both sides

If you were a judge in a case involving even a small amount of money, you wouldn't take anything as proved without a witness. A witness's word would count for nothing unless it were sworn in. You would allow both sides to be heard, and you would allow them time. You wouldn't dismiss the hearing after one sitting, because the truth will appear clear after a few sessions.

Do you condemn your friend offhand? Are you angry with him before you hear his story? Before you have questioned him? Before he knows who said what about him?

Now, have you already listened to both sides? The same person who has informed against your friend will say no more if he is obliged to prove what he says. He will say, "Don't call me as a witness; if you do, I'll deny it. Unless you don't call me, I will never tell you anything."

While he stirs up trouble for you, he withdraws himself from the strife and battle. The man who will tell you nothing except in secret doesn't tell you anything at all.

What can be more unjust than to believe a story told in secret, and to be angry about it publicly?

Think about this

We shouldn't be quick to believe what others tell us. Some people lie to deceive us, and others say things because they themselves are deceived.

CHAPTER 30

No Reason to be Angry

Key points of this chapter

1. *Anyone can offend us, from an innocent child to a powerful king.*
2. *No matter who the offender is, there is no justification for us to get angry.*

No reason to get angry

Some things we see for ourselves. In these cases, let's examine the nature and intention of the offender.

- Maybe it is a child; let us pardon the child for it cannot tell right from wrong.
- Maybe he is our father; he had been so helpful in the past that he has won the right even to wrong us, or maybe what offends him is his merit.

- Maybe it is a woman. Well, she made a mistake. Maybe it was a man who forced her to do it. What just person can be angry for something done under compulsion?
- Maybe you hurt him. There is no harm in suffering the pain which you were the first to inflict.
- Maybe your opponent is a judge. Then you should trust his opinion rather than your own.
- Maybe he is a king. Then, if he punishes you when you are guilty, yield to justice; if he punishes you when you are the innocent, yield to fate.
- Maybe it is a dumb animal or someone as stupid as a dumb animal. If you are angry with it, you will make yourself like it.
- Maybe it is a disease or a misfortune. It will affect you less if you bear it quietly.
- Maybe it is a god. Then you waste your time by being angry with him as if you want him to be angry with someone else.
- Maybe it is a good person who has wronged you. Don't believe it.
- Maybe it is a bad person. Don't be surprised. He will pay the penalty he owes you to someone else. Besides, he has already punished himself by being the offender.

Think about this

Maybe it is a good person who has wronged you. Don't believe it. Maybe it is a bad person. Don't be surprised.

CHAPTER 31

Dealing with Unfairness

Key points of this chapter

1. *We get angry when we think we are harmed or mistreated.*
2. *To avoid getting angry about things that happen, expect for anything to happen.*
3. *The power to harm is hateful. We should not hurt other human beings or animals.*
4. *Use punishment to prevent harm. Don't use it for retribution.*

Two conditions that produce anger

As I have said, two conditions produce anger:

1. We think we have been wronged. I've already discussed this in detail.
2. We think we have been mistreated. I will address this topic here.

People think some things are unfair because they shouldn't have to suffer them or because they were unexpected.

Because we believe that unforeseen things are unacceptable, we are particularly upset by them. Therefore, the most trivial stuff at home irritates us, and this is why we see treat our friends' carelessness as intentional.

We accept our indulgences, not those of others

Our challenger asks, "Why are we then upset by the injuries inflicted by our enemies?"

It is because we don't expect those particular wrongs or don't expect them on such a scale. This thinking is the result of our excessive self-love. We think that we should not be injured even by our enemies.

Each of us feels that we are monarchs. We are willing to indulge in excesses, but we are unwilling to submit to them. What makes us angry is either ignorance or arrogance.

What is there to wonder if bad people commit harmful acts? What is new about your enemy hurting you, your friend quarreling with you, your son going wrong, or your servant doing something offensive?

Fabius used to say that the most shameful excuse a general could make was, "I did not think." I believe it is the most shameful excuse that anyone can make.

Think of everything. Expect everything.

Even with people of good character, something rough will crop up. Human nature produces minds that are treacherous, ungrateful, greedy, and impious. When you are forming a judgment about someone's morals, think about the character of human beings in general.

When you are particularly happy, be particularly careful. When everything seems peaceful to you, be sure that trouble hasn't gone away. It's just lying low. Always believe that something will happen to hurt you. A sailor doesn't ever unfurl all his sails so confidently without having the tackle handy to take them in.

Power to harm is hateful and unnatural

Above all, think about this: the power to harm is detestable and unnatural to a human being whose kindness tames even wild animals. Watch how bulls yield their necks to the yoke, how elephants allow boys and women to dance on their backs unhurt, how snakes glide harmlessly over our bosoms and among our drinking cups, how within their dens bears and lions submit to be handled with complacent mouths, and wild beasts fawn upon their master. It is a shame to have exchanged habits with wild animals.

It is a crime to injure one's country. Therefore, it is also wrong to hurt one's countrymen, for everyone is a part of our country. If the whole is sacred, so must be the parts. What if the hands wished to hurt the feet? Or the eyes to hurt the hands? All our limbs are in harmony because it is in the interest of the whole body to keep each one of them safe.

Similarly, human beings should spare one another because they are born to form a society. A society, however, cannot exist unless it guards and loves all its members. We should not even destroy vipers and water-snakes and other creatures whose teeth and claws are dangerous if we could tame them as we do other animals, so they don't hurt us or others.

We shouldn't hurt other human beings or animals

If we can, we should not hurt another human being either. People should be punished, not because they have done something wrong, but to keep them from doing wrong. We should look to the future, not to the past. Punishments are acts of caution, not of anger. If everyone with a crooked and mischievous nature should be punished, no one will escape it.

Think about this

Think of everything. Expect everything. Even with people of good character, something rough will crop up.

CHAPTER 32

Don't be Eager to Avenge

Key points of this chapter

1. *We should not pay back pain with pain.*
2. *We should ignore the minor injuries we receive.*

"But anger entails some pleasure. It is sweet to pay back the pain you have suffered."

Paying back the pain received

Not at all. It is not honorable to return pain with pain. It is not like repaying one benefit with another. In the latter, it is shameful to be outdone; in the former, it is disgraceful to outdo.

People use words like revenge and retaliation. They even think they are righteous. Yet they are not much different from wrongdoers, except in the order in which they do it. The one who retaliates is excused more readily.

Noble people ignore insults

Someone who did not know Marcus Cato struck him in the public bath (Who would knowingly hurt Cato?).

When the attacker later apologized, Cato replied, "I do not remember being struck." He thought it was preferable to ignore the insult than to avenge it.

"Did the man suffer no grief for such a nerve?"

No, he received a great deal of good instead. He became acquainted with Cato. It is the mark of a great mind to view wrongs as beneath contempt.

To treat the offender as unworthy of taking revenge upon is the most disrespectful form of revenge. Many have taken slight injuries much more seriously to heart than they need by avenging them. But a great and noble person is like a large wild animal that is unmoved by the yapping of a small dog.

Think about this

It is not honorable to return pain with pain. It is not like repaying one benefit with another.

CHAPTER 33

Be Careful with the Powerful

Key points of this chapter

1. *If we use revenge as a cure, we should use it without anger.*
2. *When dealing with influential people, sometimes, we may have to bear their wrongdoing. We may even have to pretend that we are cheerful.*
3. *We pretend not to mind the wrongdoing when the powerful wrongdoer can wrong us even more.*

Our challenger says, "We are treated with more respect if we avenge our injuries."

When revenge is a cure

If we use revenge just as a remedy, let us use it without anger. Let's regard it as useful but not pleasant. Yet, it's often better to pretend not to have noticed an injury than to avenge it.

Be careful when powerful people harm you

When powerful people wrong us, not only must we bear it, but bear it cheerfully. They will do it again if they think they have succeeded in abusing us. This is the worst feature of minds that have become arrogant by prosperity. They also hate the people they have injured.

An old courtier had achieved the rare distinction of living at court until he reached old age. Someone asked him how he managed to do it. He replied:

"By accepting injuries and returning thanks for them."

Caesar's cruelty

It is often inconvenient to avenge our wrongs, and, at times, it is not even convenient to acknowledge them. Gaius Caesar, offended by the smart clothes and well-groomed hair of the son of Pastor, a distinguished Roman knight, sent him to prison. The father begged him not to harm his son. As if this reminded him of additional punishment, Gaius Caesar immediately ordered him to be executed.

Yet, so it didn't appear that his actions were brutal towards the father, he invited him to dinner on the same day. Pastor came, and his face showed no trace of ill will. Caesar put a glass of wine before him to toast his health and stationed a guard to watch him. The father went through his part, feeling as though he was drinking his son's blood. The emperor sent him perfumed oil and garlands and had him watched to see if he took them up. He did so.

On the same day he had buried his son—or rather, on the same day he had not even had the chance to bury his son—he sat down as one of the hundred guests. The gouty older man was reclining as a guest drinking such an amount that would be inappropriate even if it is on a child's birthday.

He did not shed any tear the whole while. He did not allow his grief to show even slightly. He dined just as though he had gained his request for his son's life.

You ask me why?

He had another son.

What did Priam do in the Iliad? Did he not hide his anger and clasp the knees of Achilles? Did he not kiss the hand that dealt death, stained with the blood of his son, and dine with the killer? Yes, but there were no perfumes and garlands. With many consoling words, his fierce enemy encouraged him to eat. He did ask him to drain huge glasses of wine with a guard standing over him to see that he did it.

Father's patience

Had he only feared for his life, the father would have treated the tyrant with contempt. But love for his son kept his anger in check. He deserved the emperor's permission to leave the banquet and gather up the bones of his son. But the young Caesar, kindly and polite, would not even permit him to do this. He tormented the older man with frequent invitations to drink, advising him to lighten his sorrows.

The father, on the other hand, appeared to be in good spirits and to have forgotten what had been done that day. He would have lost his second son if he had proved an unacceptable guest to the murderer of his eldest.

Think about this

It is often inconvenient to avenge our wrongs, and, at times, it is not even convenient to acknowledge them.

CHAPTER 34

Keep Anger at a Distance

Key points of this chapter

1. *We should always keep anger at a distance.*
2. *It is the mark of the small-minded to want to retaliate all the time.*
3. *We need to forgive others because we ourselves seek forgiveness at times.*
4. *By not being angry, we can turn enemies into friends.*
5. *It takes two to fight. It is better to walk away than to retaliate.*

Keep anger at a distance

We should, therefore, keep anger at a distance. It does not matter whether the person who provokes us is our peer, our superior, or our subordinate. Conflict with one's peer will have an uncertain outcome; with one's superior, it is foolish; and with one's inferior, it is disgraceful.

The small-minded always retaliate

It is the mark of a small-minded and miserable person to try to get back at someone who snaps at him. Even mice and ants show their teeth if you lay your hand on them. All feeble creatures think that they are hurt if they are touched.

We will calm down if we recall any good the other person may have done. Let this balance his offense. Think how we will rise in others' estimation when we gain a reputation for forgiveness. Think how many people may become our valuable friends when we forgive.

We also seek forgiveness

Sulla's cruelty teaches us not to be angry with the children of our public or private enemies. He sent the sons of the outlawed into exile. Nothing is more unjust than someone inheriting his father's feuds.

Whenever we find it hard to forgive, let us think whether it would be to our advantage that all men should be beyond the reach of pleading. How often has someone who refuses to forgive others, in turn, sought forgiveness for himself? How often have they crawled at the feet of a person whom they rejected as their own?

Advantages of not being angry

What can be more glorious than turning anger into friendship? What allies could be more faithful to the Romans than those who have been their unbending enemies? Where would our empire be today had we not unified the conquered and the conquerors?

It takes two to fight

If anyone is angry with you, meet their anger by returning benefits. Fights cease when there is only one party because it takes two to fight. What if there is a bitter struggle on both sides? Even then, the one who walks away is a better person. The winner is the real loser.

Someone hit you. Do you hit back? If you do, you allow the other person to hit you again. You will not be able to withdraw from the fight when you want.

Think about this

Someone hit you. Do you hit back? If you do, you allow the other person to hit you again. You will not be able to withdraw yourself from the fight when you want.

CHAPTER 35

Anger is Ugly

Key points of this chapter

1. *Anger doesn't care if it hurts itself.*
2. *Anger is not easy to control. Anger is ugly, and it makes us look ugly.*

Would you strike an enemy so that you hurt your own hand and lose your balance? Yet, anger is such a weapon. It can only be withdrawn with difficulty. When we choose weapons, we want them to be handy and manageable. Shouldn't we avoid the clumsy, unwieldy, and irreversible?

Anger is not easy to control

The only speed you should find acceptable is the one you can stop when you want it. It should go no farther from your goal, and you should make it walk, not run. We know our muscles are diseased when they start twitching against our will. You must be old or weak if you run when you mean to walk. The healthiest and soundest movements of the mind are those that are under our control and not those out of our control.

Anger makes us look ugly

The angry have no grace left in them. They may wear fashionable clothes, but they will let them trail on the ground and won't care how they look. Their hair may be arranged well either naturally or by design, and yet it will bristle wildly, along with their mind. Their veins swell, their chest shakes by rapid breathing, their necks bulge as they shout frantically. Their limbs tremble, their hands are restless, their entire body sways back and forth.

What do you think is the state of mind of someone whose outward appearance is so shocking? How much more terrifying should their internal state be when their breathing is so rough, and their anger is so focused that it would burst unless they vent it?

Let's paint anger looking like wild animals dripping with blood or like those who are going to kill them; like the monsters, encircled with serpents, breathing fire as poets imagined; like their issuing orders to kindle war among nations and destroy peace. Let's paint anger with eyes blazing, voice hissing, roaring, grating, and making any noise that is even more terrifying, brandishing weapons in both hands without even protecting itself, gloomy, bloody, bruised with self-inflicted wounds, reeling like a maniac, wrapped in a thick cloud, running around everywhere, spreading misery and panic. Everyone— including itself—loathes it. If it cannot hurt its enemy, it is willing to destroy everything: earth, sea, and heaven. It is harmful and hateful at the same time.

Or, if you prefer, let us take it to be what the poets described:

There with her blood-stained scourge, Bellona fights,
And Discord in her riven robe delights.

Or let us invent an even more dreadful image for this hideous passion.

Think about this

The angry have no grace left in them.

CHAPTER 36

Anger Leads to Insanity

Key points of this chapter

1. *When we are angry, our appearance becomes ugly.*
2. *Anger has many unpleasant consequences and it quickly leads to insanity.*

When you're angry look in a mirror

Sextius says that some angry people have benefited by looking in a mirror. They have been taken aback by such a significant change in the way they look. It is as if they were brought into their own presence and could not recognize themselves.

Still, how small a part of the real ugliness of anger is reflected in the image in the mirror!

Anger has an ugly outward appearance

If the [angry] mind could be made to appear as a material, we would be baffled when we see how black and stained, how seething, twisted, and swollen it looked. Even now, when we see it through the screens of blood, bones, and so forth, it looks hideous. What would it be, were it to be seen in the open, laid bare?

You say that you don't believe that anyone would be scared by the image in the mirror. Why not? Because when an angry person comes to the mirror, he has changed it already. Angry people find no face to be fairer looking than one that is fierce and savage. This is how they want to look.

Anger harms oneself

We should rather consider how many people anger has injured by itself. In their excessive heat, some people have burst blood vessels. Some have vomited because they have strained their voices too much. Some have blurred their vision when weeping forced water into their eyes too quickly. Some have fallen sick once the fit of anger passed off.

No path leads to insanity more quickly

No road leads to madness more quickly. Many who have always been in the grip of rage have lost their reason and could never regain it. Ajax was driven mad by anger and driven to suicide by madness.

Angry people curse their children with death, reduce themselves to poverty, ruin their households. They deny they are angry like mad people deny that they are insane. They are enemies to their best friends and should be avoided by their nearest and dearest.

Regardless of laws, unless they use it to cause harm, they are stirred by the slightest provocation. They are unwilling to listen to their friends. They are violent in their actions, ready to do battle as well as be destroyed by it. All this because they are seized by the greatest evil, one that surpasses all vices.

Anger is the most powerful of passions

Other passions gain a footing in our minds little by little but anger acts suddenly and all at once. It makes all other passions obey it. It overcomes the warmest love. That's why people have killed their loved ones and embraced the one they killed.

Greed may be the toughest and unbending of passions. Yet it is trampled underfoot by anger. Anger forces greed to squander its carefully collected wealth and set fire to its house and all its possessions.

Haven't even the most ambitious people thrown away the most highly valued symbols of office? Haven't they refused honors offered to them? There is no passion that anger does not rule over.

Think about this

Other passions gain a footing in the mind little by little but anger acts suddenly and all at once. It makes all other passions obey it. It overcomes the warmest love.

The Stoic Book of Anger: Volume 2

STRATEGIES FOR DEALING WITH ANGER

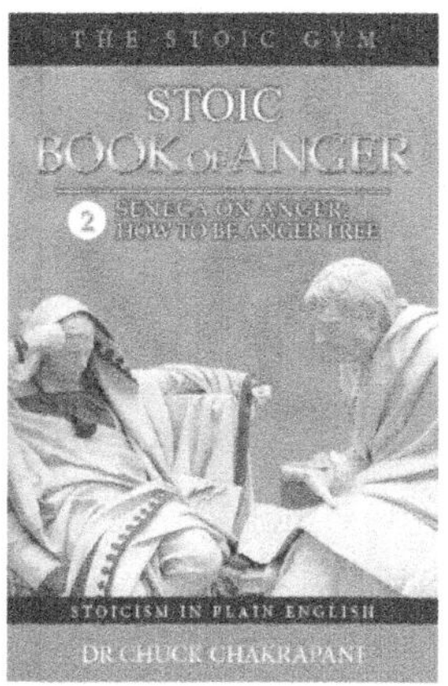

I. WHY AVOID ANGER?

- Anger is Destructive
- Anger is Unrelenting
- Anger is Useless
- Anger is Ugly
- Anger is Universal

II. HOW TO STOP ANGER ARISING

- Great Minds Avoid Anger
- Don't Attempt Too Much
- Associate with the Peaceful
- Avoid Exhaustion
- Act Quickly on Symptoms
- Don't Listen to Gossip
- Don't Act When You're Angry
- Change Signs of Anger

III. EXAMPLES TO AVOID

- King Cambyses
- The King of Persians

- King Darius
- Emperor Alexander
- Gaius Caesar
- Anger's Ferocity
- Rushing to Act Unprepared
- Waging War Against Things

IV. EXAMPLES TO FOLLOW

- Be Gentle
- Be Gracious

V. ANGER-HANDLING STRATEGIES

- See it From the Other Person's Point of View
- Tolerate Others' Faults
- Be Understanding of Others
- Heal, Don't Avenge, an Injury
- Stop Finding New Targets
- Stop Being Upset by Trifles
- Avoid Comparisons
- Be Grateful
- Use Different Approaches to Control Anger
- Beware of Money
- Beware of Trivial Things
- Beware of Your Senses
- Beware of Your Mind
- Beware of Perceived Slights
- Beware of Arrogant People
- Use a Ruse
- Don't Use Anger to Cure Anger
- The Anger-free are Peaceful
- Think About Your Mortality
- Live With Urgency

FREE DIGITAL MAGAZINE

THE STOIC: The Journal of the Stoic Gym

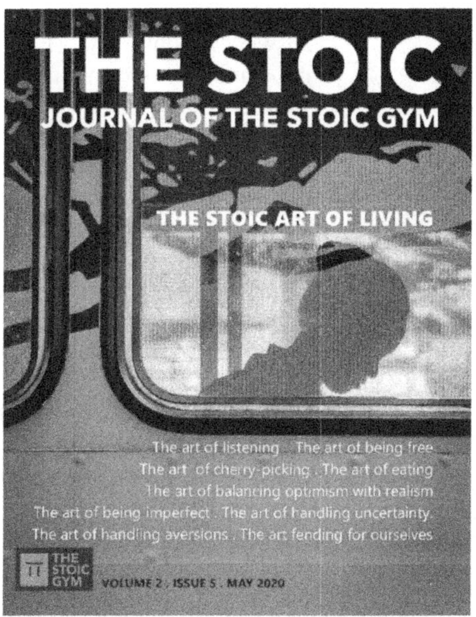

"The only magazine I read from cover to cover."

THE STOIC is the official online magazine of The Stoic Gym. It is an applied magazine designed to bring high-quality articles on how to live a life of happiness, serenity, and freedom using Stoic principles. By subscribing, you can have the magazine delivered to your inbox, as soon as an issue is published. Subscribe. It's FREE! https://www.thestoicgym.com/the-stoic-subscribe/

TWO FREE E-BOOKS

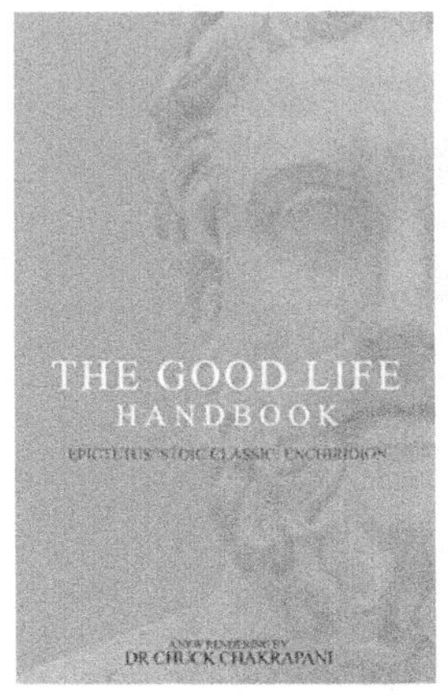

THE GOOD LIFE HANDBOOK The Handbook is a guide to the good life. It answers the question, "How can we be good and live free and happy, no matter what else is happening around us?"
"An inspiring read and one I plan to go back to whenever I need a little reminder that I can only control what I do, not what the world around me does." Elizabeth (Goodreads)
"This contemporary-language paraphrase of the Enchiridion is much more accessible than other translations I have read. .. I was pleased to find what I was looking for - an Enchiridion readable enough to give to teenagers, still true to the ideas in the book." Heather Jones
"I think this is my favorite version of the Enchiridion. Chuck has done a fantastic job here, in my opinion." Brendad Sonichsen
"Life-changing. Read it once, and you'll read it ten more times." Brandon Shinault
Ebook is available FREE at online book stores like Amazon.
https://amzn.to/2XMjpcP

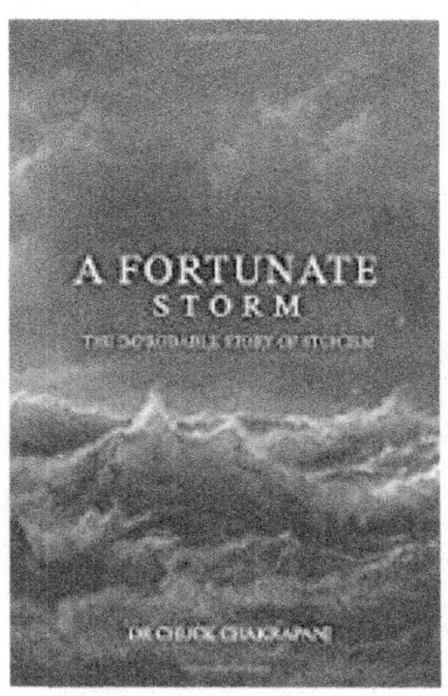

A FORTUNATE STORM Strange is the story of Stoicism. Three unconnected events – a shipwreck in Piraeus, a play in Thebes, and the banishment of a rebel in Turkey – connected three unrelated individuals to give birth to a philosophy. It was to endure two thousand years and offer hope and comfort to hundreds of thousands of people along the way. Stoicism had seven formal leaders or "scholarchs," but much of what we know of Stoicism today comes from four Stoics who lived after the all the scholarchs were gone. This is the story of those eleven people. Many others contributed to Stoicism, but to make this brief and readable, Dr. Chuck Chakrapani tells the story of Stoicism through these eleven leading figures of Stoicism. https://www.thestoicgym.com/fortunatestormfree/

UNSHAKABLE FREEDOM

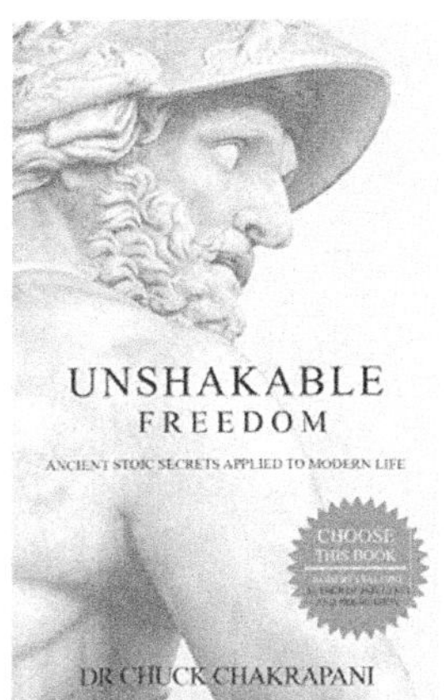

THE STOIC GUIDE TO A LIFE THAT FLOWS WELL

How can we achieve total personal freedom when we have so many obligations and so many demands on our time? Is personal freedom even possible? Yes, said the Stoics, and gave us a blueprint for freedom. Dr. Chakrapani brings their teachings to the digital era.

You'll "probably get through it in a few hours, enjoy the whole thing, and come away with an accurate and workable idea of Stoic philosophy. So please do just go and read it.
DONALD ROBERTSON, Book Reviews—Stoicism
If you want to apply [the Stoic principles] right away, it is a wonderful book for that. This will help a lot of people. This is a gateway book. Dr. GREGORY SADLER, Sadler's Honest Book Reviews.
Dr. Chakrapani has written a superbly helpful book."
BROGA, Amazon (UK)
The absolute best book by far ... is Unshakable Freedom by Chuck Chakrapani ... It explains Stoicism in an extremely accessible and easy to understand format. Highly recommended." ILLEGALUTURN, reddit/r/stoicism

Get your copy now: https://amzn.to/3dQi8Hl

HOW TO BE A STOIC WHEN YOU DON'T KNOW HOW

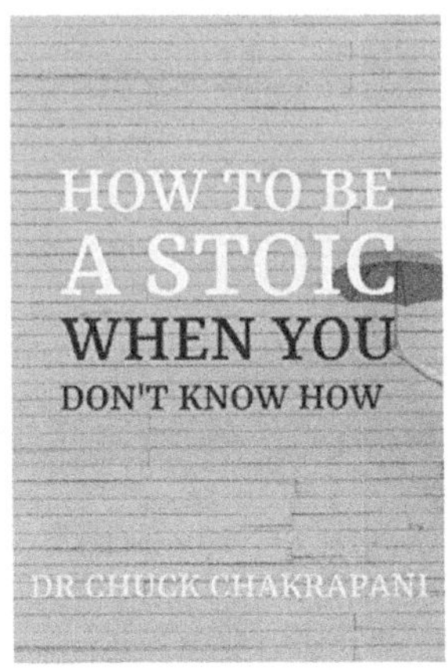

A UNIQUE 10-WEEK COURSE IN STOICISM

To help those who would like to understand and practice the fundamentals of Stoicism, The Stoic Gym has put together a unique 10-week self-study training course carefully designed to teach the essence of Stoicism. Each week's lesson starts with a big idea, followed by a discussion of how it works in practice, supported by a Stoic exercise to reinforce it, and a Stoic quote.

By the time you finish the course, you should have a solid understanding of the foundations of Stoicism. You will know how your judgments create all your problems, how to avoid them by living in accordance with nature, how to use the principle of dichotomy to live effectively, why you need to practice the four virtues—wisdom, justice, moderation, and courage—and how to practice the three disciplines: assent, desire, and action. You will know how to apply what you have learned to your daily life. This course was very carefully designed by The Stoic Gym to enable you to learn all the fundamentals quickly and easily.

Get your copy of the course today! https://amzn.to/3dQWP8z

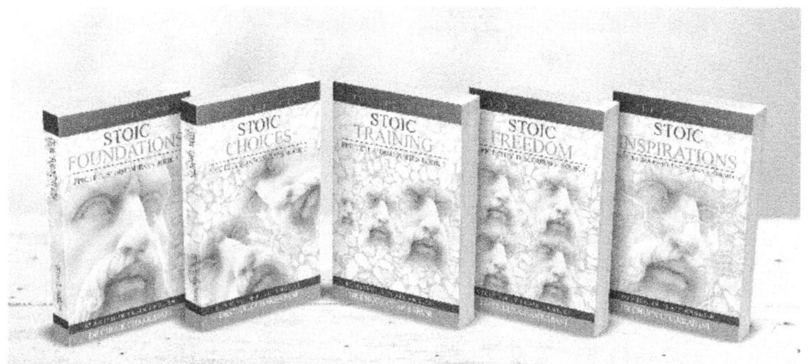

THE COMPLETE WORKS OF EPICTETUS

A SET OF FIVE INDISPENSABLE BOOKS

STOIC FOUNDATIONS (Discourses Book 1) explains the basic tenets of Stoicism. If you are interested in Epictetus' teachings, this where you should start.

STOIC CHOICES is the plain English version of Discourses Book 2. It discusses what our choices are in life and how to make better choices.

STOIC TRAINING is the third book of Discourses of Epictetus in plain English. Stoics did not only believe in theoretical knowledge but held it as critical that we practice what we learned.

STOIC FREEDOM (Discourses Book 4) focuses on freedom. Personal freedom is close to Epictetus' heart, and his rhetoric shines when he talks about it. But what does a free person look like?

STOIC INSPIRATIONS includes a summary (or extracts) from the above four books by Arrian (Enchiridion) and The Golden Sayings of Epictetus. It also includes "fragments" (quotes) as well as a biography.

Available in print and digital editions from Amazon at https://amzn.to/2YjEM4d

THE COMPLETE WORKS OF MARCUS AURELIUS (2

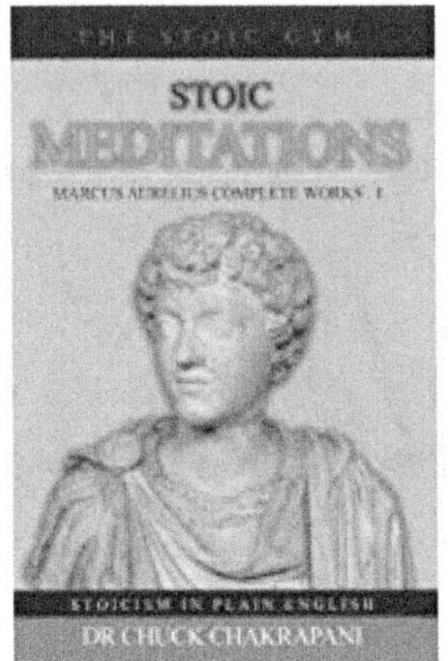

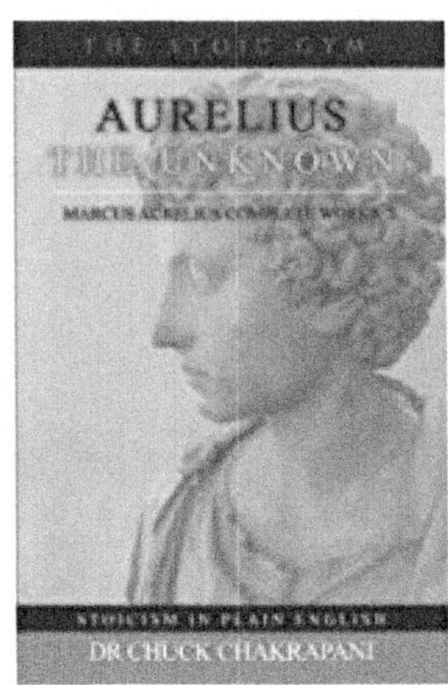

VOLS)

STOIC MEDITATIONS AURELIUS THE UNKNOWN

STOIC MEDITATIONS. *Meditations* is a classic and beloved work of Stoicism. It is the personal journal kept by the beloved Roman Emperor Marcus Aurelius. It was never meant for publication, and yet, after his death, it has become probably the most widely read book on Stoic philosophy. Meditations is a profoundly moving personal journal that is uplifting and refreshing. *Meditations* was never meant for publication, and yet it became probably the most widely read book on Stoicism. https://amzn.to/2Uv7qyt

AURELIUS THE UNKNOWN. While Meditations is one of the best-read Stoic books, not many of us know about Marcus' other writings: his personal letters and speeches. For the first time ever, *Aurelius, the Unknown* presents all his letters and speeches in a single volume. This book also includes a biographic sketch and several anecdotes from his life. A must-read for all fans of Marcus Aurelius. Much of the material is not widely available. Probably for the first time in 100 years, we present the little works of, and anecdotes about, Marcus Aurelius. So, if you are curious about Marcus Aurelius, the man (as opposed to Marcus Aurelius philosopher-king), you should read this book. https://amzn.to/3hbPSBe

THE COMPLETE WORKS OF MUSONIUS RUFUS

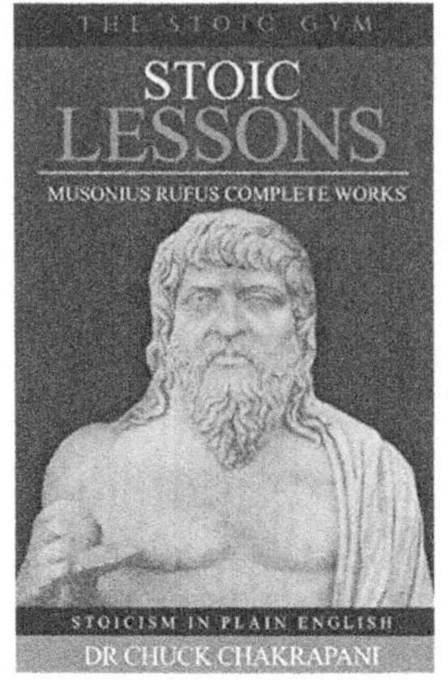

STOIC LESSONS. This is the complete works of Musonius Rufus (25-95CE), the man who taught Epictetus. While he was very well-known and respected during his time, he is less widely known now. He was a social activist, a proto-feminist, a vegetarian, and a minimalist. No topic is too small or too big for him. Here are some of the topics covered in this book: *Women and men are equal. Why are the hardships of little importance? Why should everyone study philosophy? Where you live or are forced to live is of no importance. Don't take things personally and be personally insulted. Live "according to nature" Live a virtuous family life. Live a simple life. Children should obey their parents, but not indiscriminately. If you keep practicing virtue, you don't need anything unusual in your old age.* Get your copy now: https://amzn.to/2YmVgsF

YOUR GUIDE TO EVERYTHING STOIC

THE STOIC ATLAS. This short volume is an indispensable reference for modern Stoics. It covers the following topics:

The Geography of Ancient Stoicism. The Geography of Modern Stoicism. The Timeline of Ancient Stoicism. The Timeline of Modern Stoicism. Stoicism in Words, Pictures, and Numbers. The History of Ancient Stoicism. The History of Modern Stoicism. An Outline of Ancient Stoicism. An Outline of Modern Stoicism with pictures of Stoic sites (both ancient and modern) and photographs of the Modern Stoic movement

Both the online and the print editions are in full color, beautifully produced. Get your copy https://amzn.to/2Ylzwgy

THE COMPLETE WORKS OF SENCA (In progress)

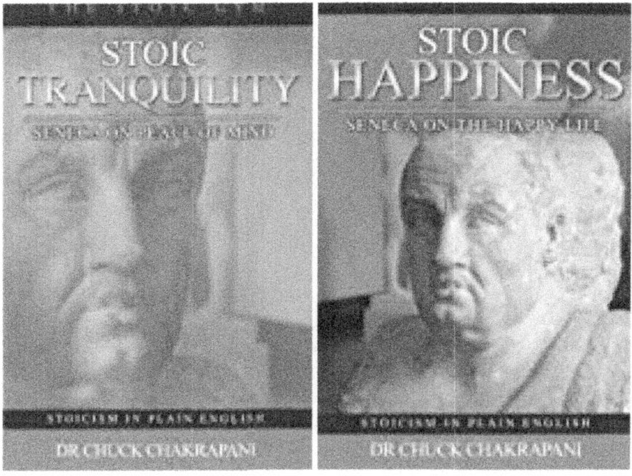

STOIC HAPPINESS. "*If you want to be happy, don't follow the crowd,*" warns Seneca, one of the best exponents of Stoicism. Seneca was concerned about applying Stoicism to everyday life. **Topics covered**: *How can we make Stoicism work for us, so we can live happily, fearlessly, and peacefully? In this short book addressed to his brother, Seneca addresses the problem of happiness. What are the basics of happiness? What is the path to happiness?* How to use pleasure and not be used by it?* Why should we ignore criticism and pursue virtue?* How to enjoy the wealth that comes our way and not be a slave to it?* Get your copy today: *https://amzn.to/2XNitVR*

STOIC TRANQUILITY. Seneca's advice on how to be peaceful, no matter what happens in life. In this gentle book, Seneca explains how to achieve a tranquil life. **Contents**. *Why We Are Restless. Be Alive Until You Die. Match Your Tasks With Your Ability. Be Careful in Choosing a Friend. Don't go After Possessions. Avoid Excess. Handle Life With Skill. Foresee Adversity. Avoid Useless Activity. Be Prepared for Disappointments. Avoid Stubbornness and Indecision. Take a Lighter View of Thingswhen Bad Things Happen to Good People. Relax, Practice Moderation, and Be Vigilant*. Get your copy today: *https://amzn.to/2XNitVR*

THE COMPLETE WORKS OF SENCA (In progress)

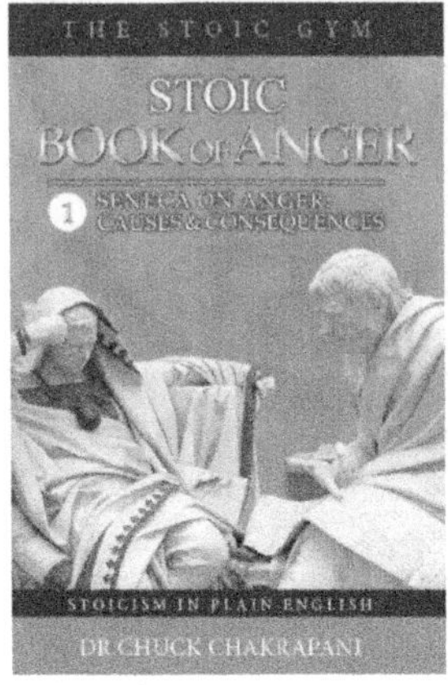

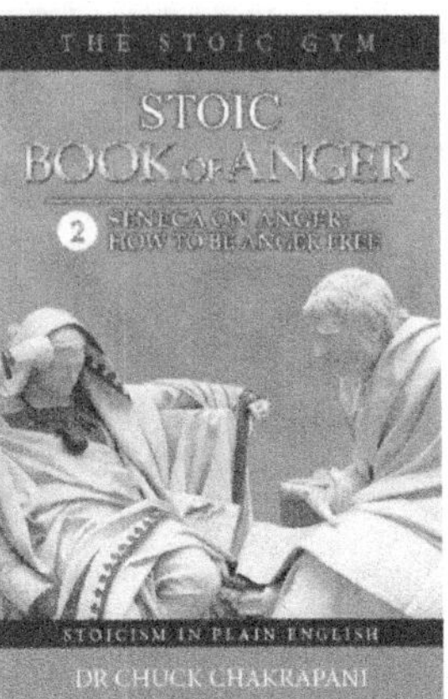

THE STOIC BOOK OF ANGER (IN 2 VOLUMES)

PROBABLY THE BEST BOOK EVER WRITTEN ON ANGER

In these two volumes, Seneca sets out to explain how we may live a life that is totally free of anger.

STOIC BOOK OF ANGER, VOLUME 1. In this volume, Seneca sets the stage for an anger-free life. He explores the causes and consequences of anger: Why do we get angry? Do we choose to be angry, or is it thrust upon us by nature? How do we look when we are angry? How do mental habits stoke anger? What can we do about it? Can anger be helpful -ever? Is it ever possible to get get rid of anger entirely from our lives?

STOIC BOOK OF ANGER, VOLUME 2. Here, Seneca starts by reviewing why anger is destructive and why we should stop it from arising. He then provides several historical examples for us to follow and avoid. Finally, he gives several specific anger handling strategies. Seneca's insights into anger are so deep, and his anger management techniques are so powerful that they are still being used by modern psychotherapies such as Cognitive Behavior Therapy.

About the Author

This book is a plain English version of the Stoic philosopher Seneca's On Anger or *De Ira.* This modern version is authored by Dr. Chuck Chakrapani.

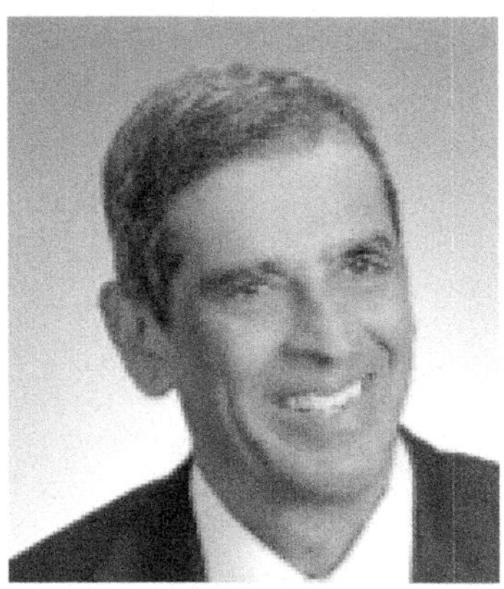

Chuck, the editor of THE STOIC magazine, is a psychologist by training, a data scientist by profession, and a Stoic author by choice. He is the president of Leger Analytics, Distinguished Visiting Professor at Ryerson University, and the Chief Knowledge Officer of the Blackstone Group in Chicago.

Chuck is a prolific writer and has written over 30 books and 500 articles on different subjects ranging from investment strategies, marketing research, psychology, Statistics, analytics, to Stoicism.

He can be reached at TheStoic@TheStoicGym.com

Made in United States
North Haven, CT
25 April 2024

51766761R10136